SIRTFOOL

GET THEM SKINNY GENES

The Vegetarian Low-Calorie Fast Metabolism Diet for Weight Loss

Elian Stephens

Copyright © 2020 Elian Stephens

All Rights Reserved

Copyright 2020 By Elian Stephens - All rights reserved.

The following book is produced below with the goal of providing information that is as accurate and reliable as possible. Regardless, purchasing this eBook can be seen as consent to the fact that both the publisher and the author of this book are in no way experts on the topics discussed within and that any recommendations or suggestions that are made herein are for entertainment purposes only. Professionals should be consulted as needed prior to undertaking any of the action endorsed herein.

This declaration is deemed fair and valid by both the American Bar Association and the Committee of Publishers Association and is legally binding throughout the United States.

Furthermore, the transmission, duplication or reproduction of any of the following work including specific information will be considered an illegal act irrespective of if it is done electronically or in print. This extends to creating a secondary or tertiary copy of the work or a recorded copy and is only allowed with express written consent from the Publisher. All additional right reserved.

The information in the following pages is broadly considered to be a truthful and accurate account of facts and as such any inattention, use or misuse of the information in question by the reader will render any resulting actions solely under their purview. There are no scenarios in which the publisher or the original author of this work can be in any fashion deemed liable for any hardship or damages that may befall them after undertaking information described herein.

Additionally, the information in the following pages is intended only for informational purposes and should thus be thought of as universal. As befitting its nature, it is presented without assurance regarding its prolonged validity or interim quality. Trademarks that are mentioned are done without written consent and can in no way be considered an endorsement from the trademark holder.

Table of Contents

PART I 11

Sirtfood Diet 12

    Chapter 1: Health Benefits of the Diet 12

    Chapter 2: Sirtfood Juice Recipes 14

        Green Juice 15

        Blueberry Kale Smoothie 16

        Tropical Kale Smoothie 17

        Strawberry Oatmeal Smoothie 18

    Chapter 3: Main Course Recipes for Sirtfood Diet 19

        Green Juice Salad 19

        King Prawns and Buckwheat Noodles 20

        Red Onion Dhal and Buckwheat 22

        Chicken Curry 24

        Chickpea Stew With Baked Potatoes 27

        Blueberry Pancakes 29

        Sirtfood Bites 31

        Flank Steak With Broccoli Cauliflower Gratin 33

        Kale Celery Salad 36

        Buckwheat Stir Fry 38

        Kale Omelet 40

        Tuna Rocket Salad 41

        Turmeric Baked Salmon 43

    Chapter 4: One-Week Meal Plan 45

PART II 47

Chapter 1: Health Benefits of the Hormone Diet..48

Chapter 2: Hormone-Rebalancing Smoothies 51

    Estrogen Detox Smoothie..51

    Dopamine Delight Smoothie..53

    Breakfast Smoothie Bowl..54

    Blueberry Detox Smoothie...56

    Maca Mango Smoothie 57

    Pituitary Relief Smoothie..58

Chapter 2: Easy Breakfast Recipes 59

    Scrambled Eggs With Feta and Tomatoes 59

    Smashed Avo and Quinoa..61

    Hormone Balancing Granola...62

Chapter 3: Healthy Lunch Recipes..64

    Easy Shakshuka 64

    Ginger Chicken 66

    Carrot and Miso Soup...67

    Arugula Salad 69

    Kale Soup 71

    Roasted Sardines 72

Chapter 4: Tasty Dinner Recipes 74

    Rosemary Chicken...75

    Corned Beef and Cabbage..76

    Roasted Parsnips and Carrots..77

    Herbed Salmon 78

    Chipotle Cauliflower Tacos..80

PART III..82

Chapter 1: Tasty Breakfast Options..83

French Crepe 83
Chapter 2: Delicious Salads 87
   Traditional French Country Salad With Lemon Dijon Vinaigrette 87
Chapter 3: Soup 89
   Classic French Onion Bistro Soup 89
   Fresh French Pea Soup 91
   Green Vegetable Soup 93
Chapter 4: Beef Options 95
   Beef Bourguignon - Slow-Cooked 95
   Entrecote Steak With Red Wine Sauce 98
   Pan-Seared Steak au Poivre 100
   Steak Diane 102
Chapter 5: Other Delicious French Classics 104
   French Ham & Grilled Cheese Sandwich - Croque Monsieur 104
   Pork Chops With Mustard Sauce 106
   Provencal Chicken Casserole 108
   White Wine Coq Au Vin 109
PART IV 111
   Chapter 1: What Is Carnivore Diet? 112
   Chapter 2: Recipes for Tasty Appetizers 116
      Oven-Baked Chicken Wings 116
      Steak Nuggets 118
      Grilled Shrimp 120
      Roasted Bone Marrow 122
      Bacon-Wrapped Chicken Bites 123
      Salami Egg Muffins 124

3-Ingredients Scotch Eggs..125

Chapter 3: Quick and Easy Everyday Recipes 127

Carnivore Waffles..127

Chicken Bacon Pancakes..128

Garlic Cilantro Salmon 129

Mustard-Seared Bacon Burgers..130

Crockpot Shredded Chicken..132

Chapter 4: Weekend Dinner Recipes 133

Organ Meat Pie 133

Smokey Bacon Meatballs...134

Steak au Poivre...135

Skillet Rib Eye Steaks..137

Pan-Fried Pork Tenderloin...138

Carnivore Chicken Enchiladas..139

PART V...141

Grilling Rub 142

Chapter 1: Seafood 144

Lemony Shrimp & Tomatoes 144

Sea Bass With Garlic Butter 146

Chapter 2: Pork... 148

Grilled Sausages With Summer Veggies..148

Honey-Chipotle Ribs...150

Peachy Pork Ribs 152

Pork Loin Steaks 154

Chapter 3: Poultry 156

Chicago-Style Turkey Dogs..156

Dr. Pepper Drumsticks 157
Grilled Lemon Chicken 158
Ground Turkey Burgers 160
Spiced Chicken With Cilantro Lime Butter 162
Turkey Pepper Kabobs 164

Chapter 4: Beef 166

Classic Beef Cheeseburgers 166
Grilled Skirt Steak With Peppers & Onions 168
Tangy Lime Top Round Steak 170
Whiskey Cheddar Burgers 171

Chapter 5: Dessert 173

Grilled Pineapple With Lime Dip 173
Take Care Of Your Grill! 175

PART VI 176

Chapter 1: Easy Recipes for Managing Kidney Problems 177

Pumpkin Pancakes 178
Pasta Salad 180
Broccoli and Apple Salad 181
Pineapple Frangelico Sorbet 183
Egg Muffins 184
Linguine With Broccoli, Chickpeas, and Ricotta 186
Ground Beef Soup 189
Apple Oatmeal Crisp 190

Chapter 2: Weekend Recipes for Renal Diet 191

Hawaiian Chicken Salad Sandwich 191
Apple Puffs 192

Creamy Orzo and Vegetables 193

Minestrone Soup 195

Frosted Grapes 197

Yogurt and Fruit Salad 198

Beet and Apple Juice Blend 200

Baked Turkey Spring Rolls 201

Crab-Stuffed Celery Logs 203

Couscous Salad 204

Chapter 3: One-Week Meal Plan 206

PART I

Sirtfood Diet

The sirtfood diet is one of the latest diet patterns that has garnered quite the attention. The idea was brought to the market by two nutritionists Glen Matten and Aidan Goggins. The main idea of the diet revolves around sirtuins, which are basically a group of 7 proteins that are responsible for the functioning and regulation of lifespan, inflammation, and metabolism (Sergiy Libert, 2013).

Chapter 1: Health Benefits of the Diet

The benefits are vast. This includes loss in weight, better skin quality, gain in muscle mass in the areas that are very much required, increased metabolic rate, feeling of fullness without having to eat much (this is the power of the foods actually), suppressing the appetite, and leading a better and confident life. This specifically includes an increase in the memory, supporting the body to control blood sugar and blood cholesterol level in a much-advanced way, and wiping out the damage caused by the free radicals and thus preventing them from having adverse impacts on the cells that might lead to other diseases like cancer.

The consumption of these foods, along with the drinks, has a number of observational shreds of evidence that link the sirtfoods with the reducing hazards of several chronic diseases. This diet is notably suited as an anti-aging scheme. Sirtfoods have the ability to satiate the appetite in a natural way and increase the functioning of the muscle. These two points are enough to find a solution that can ultimately help us to achieve a healthy weight. In addition to this, the health-improving impact of these compounds is powerful in comparison to the drugs that are prescribed in order to prevent several chronic diseases like that of diabetes, heart problems, Alzheimer's, etc.

A pilot study was conducted on a total of 39 participants. At the end of the first week, the participants had an increase in muscle mass and also lost 7 pounds on average. Research has proven that in this initial week, the weight loss that is witnessed is mostly from water, glycogen, and muscle, and only one-third of it is from fat (Manfred J. Müller, 2016). The major sirtfoods include red wine, kale, soy, strawberries, matcha green tea, extra virgin olive oil, walnuts, buckwheat, capers, lovage, coffee, dark chocolate, Medjool dates, turmeric, red chicory, parsley, onions, arugula, and blueberries (Kathrin Pallauf, 2013).

Chapter 2: Sirtfood Juice Recipes

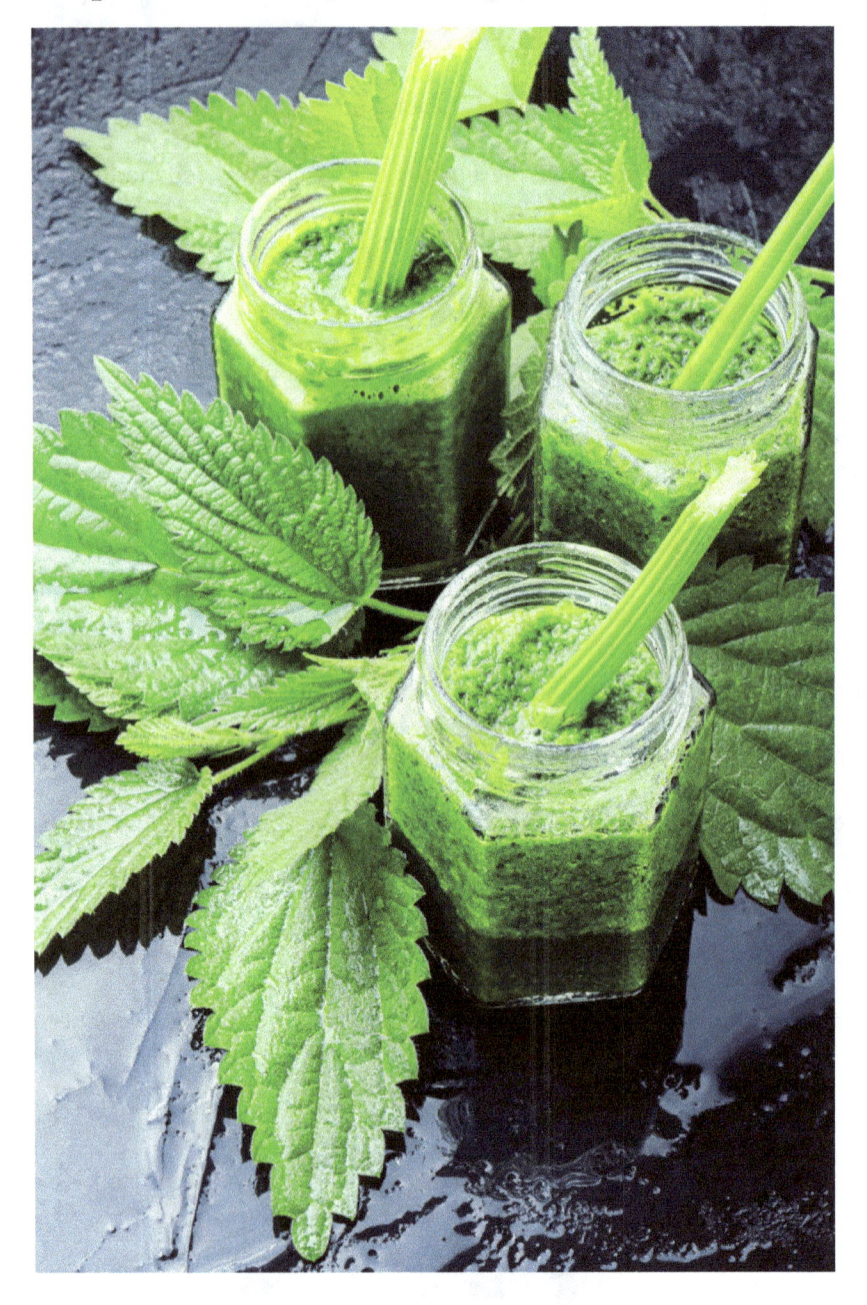

Green Juice

Total Prep & Cooking Time: Five minutes

Yields: 1 serving

Nutrition Facts: Calories: 182.3 | Carbs: 42.9g | Protein: 6g | Fat: 1.5g | Fiber: 12.7g

Ingredients:

- Half a green apple
- Two sticks of celery
- Five grams of parsley
- Thirty grams of rocket
- Seventy-five grams of kale
- Half a teaspoon of matcha green tea
- Juice of half a lemon
- One cm of ginger

Method:

1. Juice the kale, rocket, celery sticks, green apple, and parsley in a juicer.
2. Add the lemon juice into the green juice by squeezing it with your hand.
3. Take a glass and pour a little amount of the green juice into it. Add the matcha green tea and stir it in. Then, pour the remaining green juice into the glass and stir to combine everything properly.
4. You can choose to save it for later or drink it straight away.

Blueberry Kale Smoothie

Total Prep & Cooking Time: Five minutes

Yields: 1 serving

Nutrition Facts: Calories: 240 | Carbs: 37.9g | Protein: 17.2g | Fat: 3.6g | Fiber: 7g

Ingredients:

- Half a cup each of
    - Plain low-fat yogurt
    - Blueberries (frozen or fresh)
    - Kale, chopped
- Half a banana
- Half a teaspoon of cinnamon powder
- One tablespoon of flaxseed meal
- One scoop of protein powder
- Half a cup of water (optional)
- Two handfuls of ice (you can add more if you like)

Method:

1. Take a high-speed blender and add all the ingredients in it.
2. Blend everything together until you get a smooth puree.
3. Pour the blueberry kale smoothie in a glass and serve cold.

Tropical Kale Smoothie

Total Prep & Cooking Time: 10 minutes

Yields: 2 servings

Nutrition Facts: Calories: 187 | Carbs: 46.8g | Protein: 3.5g | Fat: 0.5g | Fiber: 4.7g

Ingredients:

- Half a cup to one cup of orange juice (about 120 ml to 240 ml)
- One banana, chopped (use frozen banana, is possible)
- Two cups of pineapple (about 330 grams), chopped (use frozen pineapple if possible)
- One and a half cups of kale (around 90 grams), chopped

Method:

1. Add the chopped bananas, pineapple, kale, and orange juice into a blender and blend everything together until you get a smooth puree.
2. You can add more orange juice if you need to attain a smoothie consistency. The amount of frozen fruit used directly affects the consistency of the smoothie.
3. Pour the smoothie equally into two glasses and serve cold.

Strawberry Oatmeal Smoothie

Total Prep & Cooking Time: 5 minutes

Yields: 2 servings

Nutrition Facts: Calories: 236.1 | Carbs: 44.9g | Protein: 7.6g | Fat: 3.7g | Fiber: 5.9g

Ingredients:

- Half a tsp. of vanilla extract
- Fourteen frozen strawberries
- One banana (cut into chunks)
- Half a cup of rolled oats
- One cup of soy milk
- One and a half tsps. of white sugar

Method:

1. Take a blender. Add the strawberries, banana, oats, and soy milk.
2. Then add sugar and vanilla extract.
3. Blend until the texture becomes smooth.
4. Then pour it into a glass and serve.

Chapter 3: Main Course Recipes for Sirtfood Diet

Green Juice Salad
Total Prep & Cooking Time: Ten minutes

Yields: 1 serving

Nutrition Facts: Calories: 199 | Carbs: 27g | Protein: 10g | Fat: 8.2g | Fiber: 9.2g

Ingredients:

- Six walnuts, halved
- Half of a green apple, sliced
- Two sticks of celery, sliced
- One tablespoon each of
    - Parsley
    - Olive oil
- One handful of rocket
- Two handfuls of kale, sliced
- One cm of ginger, grated
- Juice of half a lemon
- Salt and pepper to taste

Method:

1. To make the dressing, add the olive oil, ginger, lemon juice, salt, and pepper in a jam jar. Shake the jar to combine everything together.

2. Keep the sliced kale in a large bowl and add the dressing over it. Massage the dressing for about a minute to mix it with the kale properly.

3. Lastly, add the remaining ingredients (walnuts, sliced green apple, celery sticks, parsley, and rocket) into the bowl and combine everything thoroughly.

King Prawns and Buckwheat Noodles

Total Prep & Cooking Time: Twenty minutes

Yields: 4 servings

Nutrition Facts: Calories: 496 | Carbs: 53.2g | Protein: 22.2g | Fat: 17.6g | Fiber: 4.8g

Ingredients:

- 600 grams of king prawn
- 300 grams of soba or buckwheat noodles (using 100 percent buckwheat is recommended)
- One bird's eye chili, membranes, and seeds eliminated and finely chopped (and more according to taste)
- Three cloves of garlic, finely chopped or grated
- Three cm of ginger, grated
- 100 grams of green beans, chopped
- 100 grams of kale, roughly chopped
- Two celery sticks, sliced
- One red onion, thinly sliced
- Two tablespoons each of
    - Parsley, finely chopped (or lovage, if you have it)
    - Soy sauce or tamari (and extra for serving)
    - Extra virgin olive oil

Method:

1. Boil the buckwheat noodles for three to five minutes or until they are cooked according to your liking. Drain the water and then rinse the noodles in cold water. Drizzle some olive oil on the top and mix it with the noodles. Keep this mixture aside.

2. Prepare the remaining ingredients while the noodles are boiling.

3. Place a large frying pan or a wok over low heat and add a little olive oil into it. Then add the celery and red onions and fry them for about three minutes so that they get soft.

4. Then add the green beans and kale and increase the heat to medium-high. Fry them for about three minutes.

5. Decrease the heat again and then add the prawns, chili, ginger, and garlic into the pan. Fry for another two to three minutes so that the prawns get hot all the way through.

6. Lastly, add in the buckwheat noodles, soy sauce/tamari, and cook it for another minute so that the noodles get warm again.

7. Sprinkle some chopped parsley on the top as a garnish and serve hot.

Red Onion Dhal and Buckwheat

Total Prep & Cooking Time: Thirty minutes

Yields: 4 servings

Nutrition Facts: Calories: 154 | Carbs: 9g | Protein: 19g | Fat: 2g | Fiber: 12g

Ingredients:

- 160 grams of buckwheat or brown rice
- 100 grams of kale (spinach would also be a good alternative)
- 200 ml of water
- 400 ml of coconut milk
- 160 grams of red lentils
- Two teaspoons each of
    - Garam masala
    - Turmeric
- One bird's eye chili, deseeded and finely chopped (plus more if you want it extra hot)
- Two cms of ginger, grated
- Three cloves of garlic, crushed or grated
- One red onion (small), sliced
- One tablespoon of olive oil

Method:

1. Take a large, deep saucepan and add the olive oil in it. Add the sliced onion and cook it on low heat with the lid closed for about five minutes so that they get softened.

2. Add the chili, ginger, and garlic and cook it for another minute.

3. Add a splash of water along with the garam masala and turmeric and cook for another minute.

4. Next add the coconut milk, red lentils along with 200 ml of water. You can do this by filling the can of coconut milk halfway with water and adding it into the saucepan.

5. Combine everything together properly and let it cook over low heat for about twenty minutes. Keep the lid on and keep stirring occasionally. If the dhal starts to stick to the pan, add a little more water to it.

6. Add the kale after twenty minutes and stir properly and put the lid back on. Let it cook for another five minutes. (If you're using spinach instead, cook for an additional one to two minutes)

7. Add the buckwheat in a medium-sized saucepan about fifteen minutes before the curry is cooked.

8. Add lots of boiling water into the buckwheat and boil the water again— Cook for about ten minutes. If you prefer softer buckwheat, you can cook it for a little longer.

9. Drain the buckwheat using a sieve and serve along with the dhal.

Chicken Curry

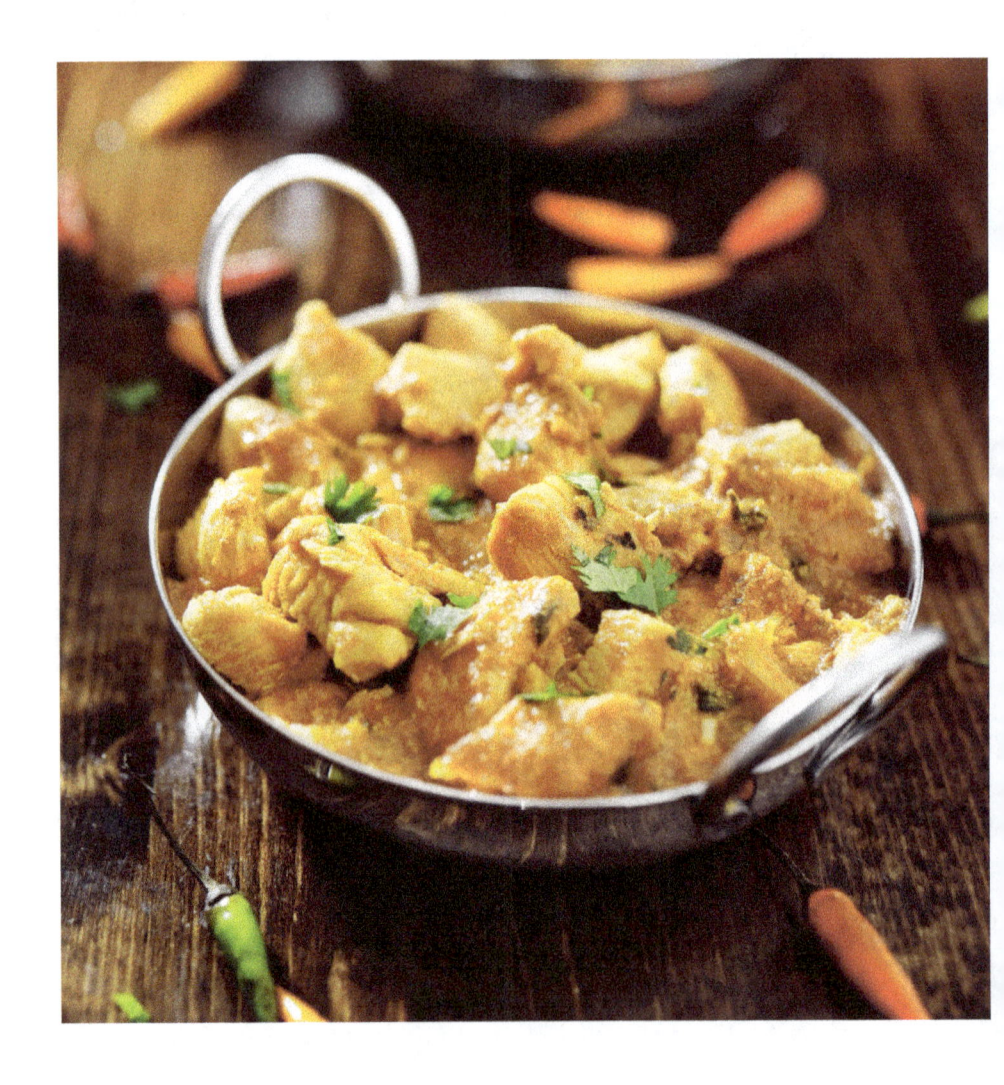

Total Prep & Cooking Time: 45 minutes

Yields: 4 servings

Nutrition Facts: Calories: 243 | Carbs: 7.5g | Protein: 28g | Fat: 11g | Fiber: 1.5g

Ingredients:

- 200 grams of buckwheat (you can also use basmati rice or brown rice)
- One 400ml tin of coconut milk
- Eight skinless and boneless chicken thighs, sliced into bite-sized chunks (you can also use four chicken breasts)
- One tablespoon of olive oil
- Six cardamom pods (optional)
- One cinnamon stick (optional)
- Two teaspoons each of
  - Ground turmeric
  - Ground cumin
  - Garam masala
- Two cm. of fresh ginger, peeled and coarsely chopped
- Three cloves of garlic, roughly chopped
- One red onion, roughly chopped
- Two tablespoons of freshly chopped coriander (and more for garnishing)

Method:

1. Add the ginger, garlic, and onions in a food processor and blitz to get a paste. You can also use a hand blender to make the paste. If you have neither, just finely chop the three ingredients and continue the following steps.

2. Add the turmeric powder, cumin, and garam masala into the paste and combine them together. Keep the paste aside.

3. Take a wide, deep pan (preferably a non-stick pan) and add one tablespoon of olive oil into it. Heat it over high heat for about a minute and then add the pieces of boneless chicken thighs. Increase the heat and stir-fry the chicken thighs for about two minutes. Then, reduce the heat and add the curry paste. Let the chicken cook in the curry paste for about three minutes and then pour half of the coconut milk (about 200ml) into it. You can also add the cardamom and cinnamon if you're using them.

4. Let it boil for some time and then reduce the heat and let it simmer for thirty minutes. The curry sauce will get thick and delicious.

5. You can add a splash of coconut milk if your curry sauce begins to get dry. You might not need to add extra coconut milk at all, but you can add it if you want a slightly more saucy curry.

6. Prepare your side dishes and other accompaniments (buckwheat or rice) while the curry is cooking.

7. Add the chopped coriander as a garnish when the curry is ready and serve immediately with the buckwheat or rice.

Chickpea Stew With Baked Potatoes

Total Prep & Cooking Time: One hour and ten minutes

Yields: 4 to 6 servings

Nutrition Facts: Calories: 348.3 | Carbs: 41.2g | Protein: 7.2g | Fat: 16.5g | Fiber: 5.3g

Ingredients:

- Two yellow peppers, chopped into bite-sized pieces (you can also use other colored bell peppers)
- Two 400-grams tins each of
    - Chickpeas (you can also use kidney beans) (don't drain the water if you prefer including it)
    - Chopped tomatoes
- Two cm. of ginger, grated
- Four cloves of garlic, crushed or grated
- Two red onions, finely chopped
- Four to six potatoes, prickled all over
- Two tablespoons each of
    - Turmeric
    - Cumin seeds
    - Olive oil
    - Unsweetened cocoa powder (or cacao, if you want)
    - Parsley (and extra for garnishing)
- Half a teaspoon to two teaspoons of chili flakes (you can add according to how hot you like things)
- A splash of water
- Side salad (optional)
- Salt and pepper according to your taste (optional)

Method:

1. Preheat your oven to 200 degrees Celsius.

2. In the meantime, prepare all the other ingredients.

3. Place your baking potatoes in the oven when it gets hot enough and allow it to cook for an hour so that they are cooked according to your preference. You can also use your regular method to bake the potatoes if it's different from this method.

4. When the potatoes are cooking in the oven, place a large wide saucepan over low heat and add the olive oil along with the chopped red onion into it. Keep the lid on and let the onions cook for five minutes. The onions should turn soft but shouldn't turn brown.

5. Take the lid off and add the chili, cumin, ginger, and garlic into the saucepan. Let it cook on low heat for another minute and then add the turmeric along with a tiny splash of water and cook it for a further minute. Make sure that the pan does not get too dry.

6. Then, add in the yellow pepper, canned chickpeas (along with the chickpea liquid), cacao or cocoa powder, and chopped tomatoes. Bring the mixture to a boil and then let it simmer on low heat for about forty-five minutes so that the sauce gets thick and unctuous (make sure that it doesn't burn). The stew and the potatoes should complete cooking at roughly the same time.

7. Finally, add some salt and pepper as per your taste along with the parsley and stir them in the stew.

8. You can add the stew on top of the baked potatoes and serve. You can also serve the stew with a simple side salad.

Blueberry Pancakes

Total Prep & Cooking Time: 25 minutes

Yields: 2 servings

Nutrition Facts: Calories: 84 | Carbs: 11g | Protein: 2.3g | Fat: 3.5g | Fiber: 0g

Ingredients:

- 225 grams of blueberries
- 150 grams of rolled oats
- Six eggs
- Six bananas
- One-fourth of a teaspoon of salt
- Two teaspoons of baking powder

Method:

1. Add the rolled oats in a high-speed blender and pulse it for about a minute or so to get the oat flour. Before adding the oats to the blender, make sure that it is very dry. Otherwise, your oat flour will turn soggy.

2. Then, add the eggs and bananas along with the salt and baking soda into the blender and blend them together for another two minutes until you get a smooth batter.

3. Take a large bowl and transfer the mixture into it. Then add the blueberries and fold them into the mixture. Let it rest for about ten minutes to allow the baking powder to activate.

4. To make the pancakes, place a frying pan on medium-high heat and add a dollop of butter into it. The butter will help to make your pancakes really crispy and delicious.

5. Add a few spoonfuls of the blueberry pancake batter into the frying pan and cook it until the bottom side turns golden. Once the bottom turns golden, toss the pancake and fry the other side.

6. Serve them hot and enjoy.

Sirtfood Bites

Total Prep & Cooking Time: 1 hour + 15 minutes

Yields: 15-20 bites

Nutrition Facts: Calories: 58.1 | Carbs: 10.1g | Protein: 0.9g | Fat: 2.3g | Fiber: 1.2g

Ingredients:

- One tablespoon each of
  - Extra virgin olive oil
  - Ground turmeric
  - Cocoa powder
- Nine ounces of Medjool dates, pitted (about 250 grams)
- One ounce (about thirty grams) of dark chocolate (85% cocoa solids), break them into pieces (you can also use one-fourth of a cup of cocoa nibs)
- One teaspoon of vanilla extract (you can also take the scraped seeds of one vanilla pod)
- One cup of walnuts (about 120 grams)
- One to two tablespoons of water

Method:

1. Add the chocolate and walnuts in a food processor and blitz them until you get a fine powder.

2. Add the Medjool dates, cocoa powder, ground turmeric, extra-virgin olive oil, and vanilla extract into the food processor and blend them together until the mixture forms a ball. Depending on the consistency of the mixture, you can choose to add or skip the water. Make sure that the mixture is not too sticky.

3. Make bite-sized balls from the mixture using your hands and keep them in the refrigerator in an airtight container. Refrigerate them for at least an hour before consuming them.

4. To get a finish of your liking, you can roll the balls in some more dried coconut or cocoa. You can store the balls in the refrigerator for up to a week.

Flank Steak With Broccoli Cauliflower Gratin

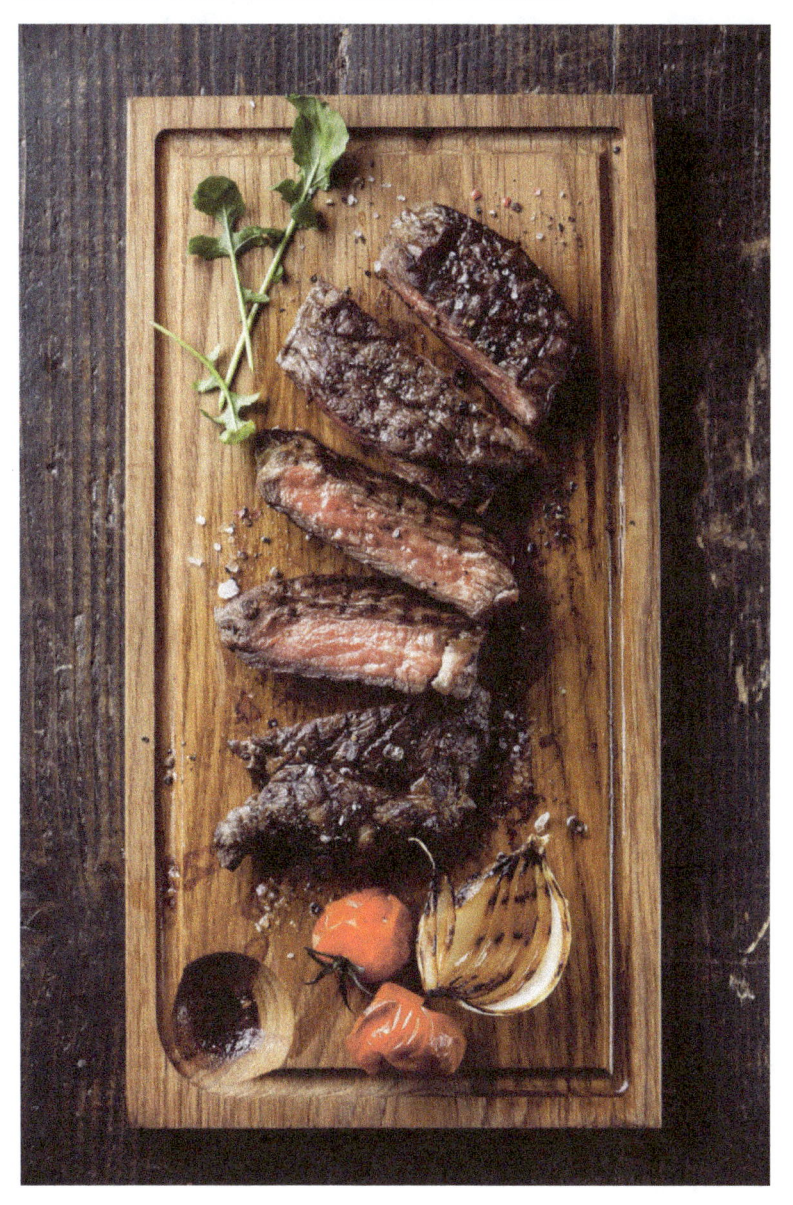

Total Prep & Cooking Time: 55 minutes

Yields: 4 servings

Nutrition Facts: Calories: 839 | Carbs: 8g | Protein: 43g | Fat: 70g | Fiber: 3g

Ingredients:

- Two tablespoons of olive oil
- Twenty ounces of flank steak
- One-fourth teaspoon salt
- Four ounces of divided shredded cheese
- Half cup of heavy whipping cream
- Eight ounces of cauliflower
- Eight ounces of broccoli
- Salt and pepper

For the pepper sauce,

- One tablespoon soy sauce
- One and a half cups of heavy whipping cream
- Half teaspoon ground black pepper

For the garnishing,

- Two tablespoons of freshly chopped parsley

Method:

1. At first, you have to preheat your oven to four hundred degrees Fahrenheit. Then you need to apply butter on a baking dish (eight by eight inches).

2. Then you have to clean and then trim the cauliflower and broccoli. Then you need to cut them into florets, and their stem needs to be sliced.

3. Then you have to boil the broccoli and cauliflower for about five minutes in salted water.

4. After boiling, you need to drain out all the water and keep the vegetables aside. Then you have to take a saucepan over medium heat and add half portion of the shredded cheese, heavy cream, and salt. Then you need to whisk them together until the cheese gets melted. Then you have to add the cauliflower and the broccoli and mix them in.

5. Place the cauliflower and broccoli mixture in a baking dish. Then you have to take the rest half portion of the cheese and add—Bake for about twenty minutes in the oven.

6. Season with salt and pepper on both sides of the meat.

7. Then you have to take a large frying pan over medium-high heat and fry the meat for about four to five minutes on each side.

8. After that, take a cutting board and place the meat on it. Then you have to leave the meat for about ten to fifteen minutes before you start to slice it.

9. Take the frying pan, and in it, you need to pour soy sauce, cream, and pepper. Then you have to bring it to a boil and allow the sauce to simmer until the sauce becomes creamy in texture. Then you need to taste it and then season it with some more salt and pepper according to your taste.

Kale Celery Salad

Total Prep & Cooking Time: 15 minutes

Yields: 4 servings

Nutrition Facts: 196 | Carbs: 20g | Protein: 5.7g | Fat: 11.5g | Fiber: 4.8g

Ingredients:

- Half a cup of crumbled feta cheese
- Half a cup of chopped and toasted walnuts
- One wedge lemon
- One red apple, crisp
- Two celery stalks
- Eight dates, pitted dried
- Four cups of washed and dried baby kale (stemmed)

For the dressing,

- Three tbsps. olive oil
- One tsp. maple syrup (or you can use any other sweetener as per your preference)
- Four tsps. balsamic vinegar
- Freshly ground salt and black pepper

Method:

1. At first, you have to take a platter or a wide serving bowl. Then you need to place the baby kale in it.

2. Cut the dates into very thin slices, lengthwise. Then you need to place it in another small bowl.

3. After that, you have to peel the celery and then cut them into halves, lengthwise.

4. Then you need to take your knife, hold it in a diagonal angle, and then cut the celery into thin pieces (approximately one to two inches each). Add these pieces to the dates.

5. Then you have to cut the sides off the apple. You need to cut very thin slices from those pieces.

6. Over the apple slices, you need to put some lemon juice to prevent them from browning.

7. For preparing the dressing, you have to take a small bowl, add maple syrup, olive oil, and vinegar. Then you need to whisk them together.

8. Once done, you have to season with freshly ground pepper and two pinches of salt.

9. Before serving, you need to take most of the dressing and pour it over the salad. Then you have to toss nicely so that they get combined. Then you need to pour the rest of the portion of the dressing over the dates and celery.

10. On the top, you have to add the date mixture, feta cheese, apple slices, and walnuts.

Buckwheat Stir Fry

Total Prep & Cooking Time: 28 minutes

Yields: 8 servings

Nutrition Facts: Calories: 258 | Carbs: 35.1g | Protein: 6.8g | Fat: 11.9g | Fiber: 2g

Ingredients:

For the buckwheat,

- Three cups of water
- One and a half cups of uncooked roasted buckwheat groats
- Pinch of salt

For the stir fry,

- Half a cup of finely chopped basil
- Half a cup of finely chopped parsley
- One teaspoon salt
- Four tablespoons of divided red palm oil or coconut oil
- Two cups of drained and chopped marinated artichoke hearts
- Four large bell peppers (sliced into strips)
- Four large minced cloves of garlic
- One bunch of finely chopped kale (ribs removed)

Method:

For making the buckwheat,

1. In a medium-sized pot, pour the buckwheat. Then rinse with cold water and drain the water. Repeat this process for about two to three times.

2. Then add three cups of water to it and also add a pinch of salt. Cover the pot and bring it to a boil.

3. Reduce the heat to low and then cook for about fifteen minutes. Keep the lid on and remove the pot from the heat.

4. Leave it for three minutes and then fluff with a fork.

For making the stir fry,

1. At first, you have to take a ceramic non-stick wok and preheat over medium heat. Then you need to add one tablespoon of oil and coat it. Then you have to add garlic and then sauté for about ten seconds. Then you need to add kale and then add one-fourth teaspoon of salt. Then you need to sauté it accompanied by occasional stirring, until it shrinks in half. Then you have to transfer it to a medium-sized bowl.

2. Then again return to the wok, turn the heat on high, and pour one tablespoon of oil. You need to add one-fourth teaspoon salt and pepper. Then you have to sauté it until it turns golden brown in color. Once done, you need to place it in the bowl containing kale.

3. Then you have to reduce the heat to low, and you need to add two tablespoons of oil. Add the cooked buckwheat and stir it nicely so that it gets coated in the oil. Then after turning off the heat, you need to add the kale and peppers, basil, parsley, artichoke hearts, and half teaspoon salt. Gently stir and serve it hot.

Kale Omelet

Total Prep & Cooking Time: 10 minutes

Yields: 1 serving

Nutrition Facts: Calories: 339 | Carbs: 8.6g | Protein: 15g | Fat: 28.1g | Fiber: 4.4g

Ingredients:

- One-fourth sliced avocado
- Pinch of red pepper (crushed)
- One tsp. sunflower seeds (unsalted)
- One tbsp. of freshly chopped cilantro
- One tbsp. lime juice
- One cup of chopped kale
- Two tsps. of extra-virgin olive oil
- One tsp. of low-fat milk
- Two eggs
- Salt

Method:

1. At first, take a small bowl and pour milk. Then you have to add the eggs and salt to it. Beat the mixture thoroughly. Then take a small non-stick skillet over medium heat, and add one tsp. of oil and heat it. Then add the egg mixture and cook for about one to two minutes, until the time you notice that the center is still a bit runny, but the bottom has become set. Then you need to flip the omelet and cook the other side for another thirty seconds until it is set too. One done, transfer the omelet to a plate.

2. Toss the kale with one tsp. of oil, sunflower seeds, cilantro, lime juice, salt, and crushed red pepper in another bowl. Then return to the omelet on the plate and top it off with avocado and the kale salad.

Tuna Rocket Salad

Total Prep & Cooking Time: 20 minutes

Yields: 4 servings

Nutrition Facts: Calories: 321 | Carbs: 20g | Protein: 33g | Fat: 12g | Fiber: 9.5g

Ingredients:

- Twelve leaves of basil (fresh)
- Two bunches of washed and dried rocket (trimmed)
- One and a half tbsps. of olive oil
- Freshly ground black pepper and salt
- Sixty grams of kalamata olives cut into halves, lengthwise (drained pitted)
- One thinly sliced and halved red onion
- Two coarsely chopped ripe tomatoes
- Four hundred grams of rinsed and drained cannellini beans
- Four hundred grams of drained tuna
- 2 cm cubes of one multigrain bread roll

Method:

1. At first, you need to preheat your oven to 200 degrees Celsius.
2. After that, take a baking tray and line it with a foil.

3. Then you have to spread the cubes of bread over the baking tray evenly.

4. Put the baking tray inside the oven and cook it for about ten minutes until it turns golden in color.

5. In the meantime, you have to take a large bowl and add the olives, onions, tomatoes, cannellini beans, and tuna. Then you need to season it with pepper and salt. Add some oil and then toss for smooth combining.

6. Your next step is to add the basil leaves, croutons, and the rocket. Then you need to toss gently to combine. After that, you can divide the salad into the serving bowls and serve.

Turmeric Baked Salmon

Total Prep & Cooking Time: 30 minutes

Yields: 4 servings

Nutrition Facts: Calories: 448 | Carbs: 2g | Protein: 34g | Fat: 33g | Fiber: 0.2g

Ingredients:

- One ripe yellow lemon
- Half a teaspoon of salt
- One teaspoon turmeric
- One tablespoon of dried thyme
- Half a cup of frozen, salted butter (you may require some more for greasing the pan)
- Four fresh one and a half inches thick salmon fillets (skin-on)

Method:

1. At first, you need to preheat your oven to 400 degrees Fahrenheit. Then with a thin layer of butter, you need to grease the bottom of the baking sheet. Rinse the salmon fillets and pat them dry. Then you have to place the salmon fillets on the buttered baking dish keeping the skin side down.

2. Take the lemons and cut them into four round slices. Remove the seeds and then cut each slice into two halves. Then you will have eight pieces.

3. Take a small dish and combine turmeric, dried thyme, and salt. Then you need to mix them well until they are nicely combined. On the top of the salmon fillets, you need to evenly sprinkle the spice mixture.

4. Place two lemon slices over each salmon fillet.

5. After that, you need to grate the cold butter on the top of the salmon fillets evenly. Allow the butter to meltdown and form a delicious sauce.

6. Then you have to cover the pan with parchment or aluminum foil. Put it inside the oven and cook for about fifteen to twenty minutes according to your desire. The cooking time is dependent on the thickness of the salmon fillets. You can check whether it is done or not by cutting into the center.

7. Once done, remove it from the oven and then uncover it. The butter sauce needs to be spooned over from the tray.

8. Top it off with fresh mint and serve.

Chapter 4: One-Week Meal Plan

Day 1

8 AM – Green Juice

12 PM - Blueberry Kale Smoothie

4 PM – Tropical Kale Smoothie

8 PM – Turmeric Baked Salmon

Day 2

8 AM – Tropical Kale Smoothie

12 PM – Green Juice

4 PM – Strawberry Oatmeal Smoothie

8 PM – King Prawns and Buckwheat Noodles

Day 3

8 AM – Strawberry Oatmeal Smoothie

12 PM – Tropical Kale Smoothie

4 PM – Green Juice

8 PM – Buckwheat Stir Fry

Day 4

8 AM – Blueberry Kale Smoothie

12 PM – Green Juice

4 PM – Green Juice Salad

8 PM – Tuna Rocket Salad

Day 5

8 AM – Green Juice

12 PM – Tropical Kale Smoothie

4 PM – Sirtfood Bites

8 PM – Chicken Curry

Day 6

8 AM – Strawberry Oatmeal Smoothie

12 PM – Green Juice

4 PM – Kale Celery Salad

8 PM – Flank Steak with Broccoli Cauliflower Gratin

Day 7

8 AM – Tropical Kale Smoothie

12 PM – Blueberry Kale Smoothie

4 PM – Kale Omelet

8 PM – Chickpea Stew with Baked Potatoes

PART II

Are you worried that your hormones are not at their optimal levels? Here is a diet that will solve your problems.

Chapter 1: Health Benefits of the Hormone Diet

When it comes to getting healthy through weight loss, there's never any shortage of fitness crazes and diets that claim to have the secret to easy and sustainable weight loss. One of the latest diet plans that have come into the spotlight is the hormone diet, which claims that people often struggle to lose weight because of their hormones.

A hormone diet is a 3-step process that spans over six weeks and is designed to synchronize your hormones and promote a healthy body through detoxification, nutritional supplements, exercise, and diet. The diet controls what you eat and informs you about the correct time to eat to ensure maximum benefits to your hormones. Many books have been written on this topic with supporters of the diet assuring people that they can lose weight quickly and significantly through diet and exercise and reset or manipulate their hormones. Although the diet has a few variations, the central idea around each is that correcting the body's perceived hormonal imbalances is the key to losing weight.

The most important benefit of a hormone diet is that it takes a solid stance on improving overall health through weight loss and promoting regular exercise as well as natural, nutritious foods. Apart from that, it also focuses on adequate sleep, stress management, emotional health, and other healthy lifestyle habits that are all essential components that people should follow, whether it's a part of a diet or not. Including a water diet, it aims towards losing about twelve pounds in the 1st phase and 2 pounds a week after that.

Hormones have an essential role in the body's everyday processes, like helping bones grow, digesting food, etc. They act as "chemical messengers," instructing the cells to perform specific actions and are transported around the body through the bloodstream.

One of the very important food items to be included in the hormone diet is salmon. Salmon is rich in omega-3 fatty acids, Docosahexaenoic acid, and Eicosapentaenoic acid (EPA). It is rich in selenium too. These help to lower your blood pressure and also reduce the level of unhealthy cholesterol in the blood. These make you less prone to heart diseases. Salmon is a rich source of healthy fat. If consumed in sufficient amounts, it provides you energy and helps you get rid of unwanted body fat. Salmon is well-known for giving fantastic weight loss results as it has less saturated fat, unlike other protein sources. Salmon is packed with vitamins like vitamin-k, E, D, and A. These are extremely helpful for your eyes, bone joints, etc. These vitamins are also good for your brain, regulation of metabolic balance, and repairing your muscles. Salmon's vitamins and omega-3 fatty acids are amazing for sharpening your mind. It also improves your memory retention power. If you consume salmon, you are less likely to develop dementia or mental dis-functions. Salmon has anti-inflammatory properties and is low in omega-6 fatty acid content (which is pro-inflammatory in nature and is present in a huge amount in the modern diet). It promotes healthy skin and gives you radiant and glowing skin. It is good for the winter because it helps you to stay warm. It also provides lubrication to your joints because of the abundant presence of essential minerals and fatty acids in it. Apart from this, some other things to include in your diet are arugula, kale, ginger, avocado, carrots, and so on.

There are almost sixteen hormones that can influence weight. For example, the hormone leptin produced by your fat cells is considered a "satiety hormone," which makes you feel full by reducing your appetite. As a signaling hormone, it communicates with the part of your brain (hypothalamus) that controls food intake and appetite. Leptin informs the brain when there is enough fat in storage, and extra fat is not required. This helps prevent overeating. Individuals who are obese or overweight generally have very high levels of leptin in their blood. Research shows that the level of leptin in obese individuals was almost four times higher than that in individuals with normal weight.

Studies have found that fat hormones like leptin and adiponectin can promote long-term weight loss by reducing appetite and increasing metabolism. It is believed that both these fat hormones follow the same pathway in the brain to manage blood sugar (glucose) and body weight (Robert V. Considine, 1996).

Simply put, the hormone diet works by helping to create a calorie deficit through better nutritional habits and exercise, which ultimately results in weight loss. It's also essential to consult a doctor before following this detox diet or consuming any dietary supplements.

Chapter 2: Hormone-Rebalancing Smoothies

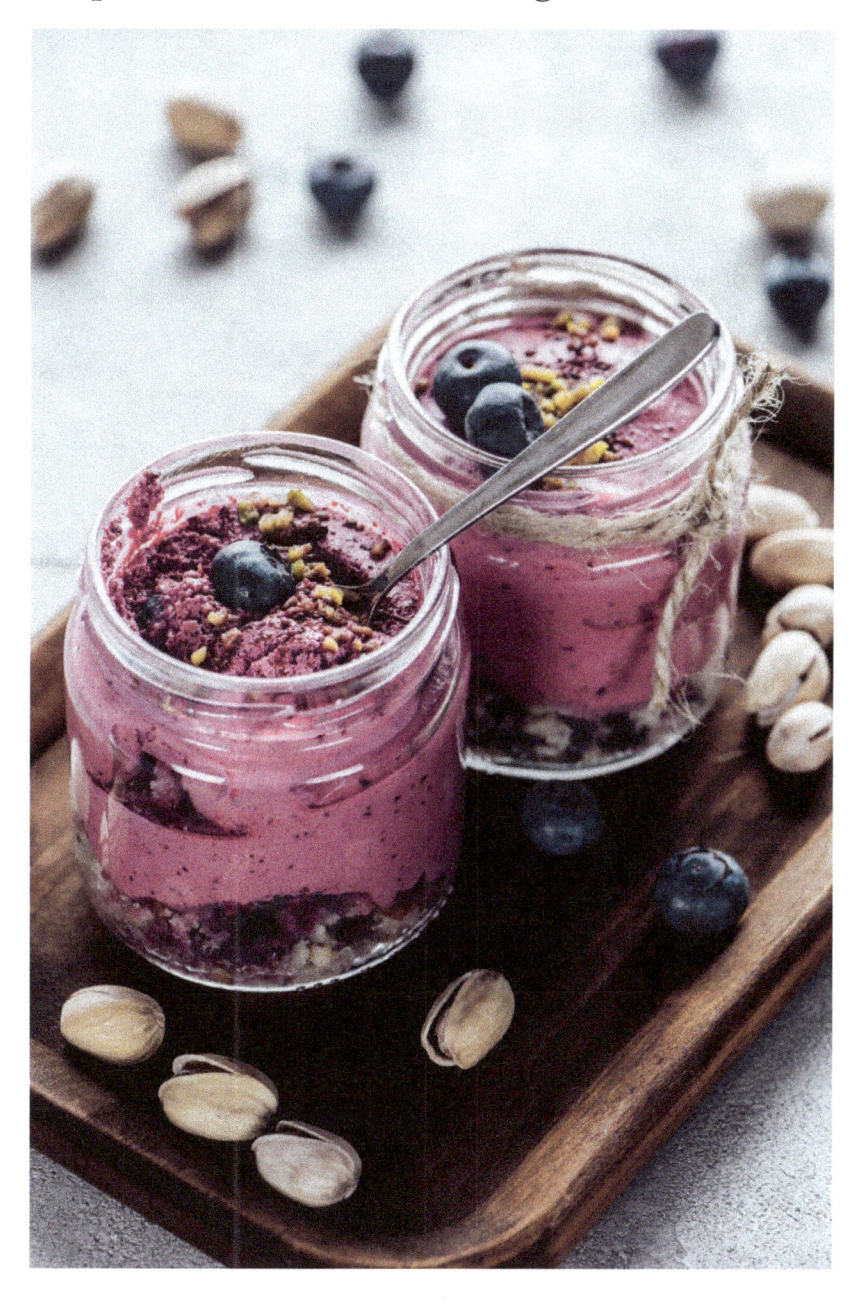

Estrogen Detox Smoothie

Total Prep & Cooking Time: 5 minutes

Yields: One glass

Nutrition Facts: Calories: 312 | Carbs: 47.9g | Protein: 18.6g | Fat: 8.5g | Fiber: 3g

Ingredients:

- Half a cup of hemp seeds
- Two kiwis (medium-sized)
- A quarter each of
  - Avocado (medium-sized)
  - Cucumber (medium-sized)
- Half a unit each of
  - Lemon (squeezed freshly)
  - Green apple
- One celery (medium-sized)
- A quarter cup of cilantro
- Two tbsps. of chis seeds
- Two cups of water (filtered)
- One tsp. of cacao nibs
- One tbsp. of coconut oil

Method:

1. Blend the ingredients all together to form a smoothie at high speed. The thickness can be adjusted according to your preference by adding more water to the mixture.

2. Serve and enjoy.

Dopamine Delight Smoothie

Total Prep Time: 10 minutes

Yields: One serving

Nutrition Facts: Calories: 383 | Carbs: 31g | Protein: 24g | Fat: 18.g | Fiber: 3g

Ingredients:

- Half a teaspoon of cinnamon (ground)
- Half a cup of peeled banana (the bananas must be frozen)
- One organic espresso, double shot (measuring half a cup)
- One tablespoon of chia seeds
- A three-fourth cup of soy milk (plain or vanilla-flavored)
- Protein powder, a serving (from the whey with the flavor of vanilla)

Method:

1. Fill in the bowl of your blender with all the ingredients (from the section of ingredients) except the whey protein powder and then proceed by switching to a high-speed blending option. Make sure it acquires a smooth consistency and then pour it out.

2. Now you may add the protein powder and give it another shot of blend until the whole things get incorporated, a bit of the goat cheese (already crumbled).

Breakfast Smoothie Bowl

Total Prep Time: 10 minutes

Yields: 2 servings

Nutrition Facts: Calories: 290 | Carbs: 53g | Protein: 6g | Fat: 8g | Fiber: 9g

Ingredients:

- One cup of thoroughly rinsed blueberries (fresh and ripe)
- A sundry of nuts and fruits for garnishing, which includes – strawberries, bananas (thinly sliced), peanuts (Spanish), kiwi (chopped), segments of tangerine, and raspberries.
- One cup of Greek yogurt

For the preparation of honey flax granola,

- Two tablespoons each of
  - Flaxseeds
  - Vegetable oil
- Oats (old-fashioned), approximately a cup
- One tablespoon of honey

Method:

1. Set your oven at a temperature of 350 degrees F.

2. Preparation of the smoothie: collect the diverse types of berries, wash them thoroughly, and then put them in the blender and turn it on. Make an even mixture out of it. Add some amount of the yogurt and blend it again to form a smooth texture.

3. For preparing the granola: Take a small-sized bowl and then drizzle a few drops oil in it. Then add the oats, flax, and honey to the oil, one by one, and mix it well. You are required to toss the bowl thoroughly to get the mixture well-coated with the poured oil. After you are done, place the oats mixture in a baking sheet evenly. Bake it for about twenty minutes. This mark will be enough to give the oats a beautiful tinge of golden brown. Allow it to cool.

4. Now you will require a shallow bowl to spoon in some yogurt, and this will be the first layer. Form a second layer with the various fruits and nuts and finally for the third layer, top with the granola.

5. Enjoy.

Notes:

- *Using frozen nuts and fruits in a warm-weather will get much to your relief.*

- *For a vegan smoothie bowl, sub the yogurt with coconut or almond yogurt.*

- *Give the pan a few strokes while baking the oats.*

Blueberry Detox Smoothie

Total Prep Time: Ten minutes

Yields: One serving

Nutrition Facts: Calories: 326 | Carbs: 65g | Protein: 4g | Fat: 8g | Fiber: 9g

Ingredients:

- One cup of wild blueberries (frozen)
- One banana (sliced into several pieces) frozen
- Orange juice (approximately half a cup)
- Cilantro leaves, fresh (approximately a measuring a small handful size)
- A quarter of an entire avocado
- A quarter cup of water

Method:

1. Add cilantro, avocado, water, blueberries, banana, and orange juice in the blender and then process.
2. Make the ingredients integrated so well that they become smooth in their consistency.

Notes: *It is recommended that you add the potent herb, cilantro, or parsley in a small amount when consuming this smoothie for the first time, as it might trigger a mild headache. If you do not get a headache, you may add a bit more of the cilantro leaves.*

Maca Mango Smoothie

Total Prep & Cooking Time: 2 minutes

Yields: 2 servings

Nutrition Facts: Calories: 53 | Carbs: 13g | Protein: 1g | Fat: 3g | Fiber: 1.5g

Ingredients:

- One and a half cups each of
    - Fresh mango
    - Frozen mango
- One tablespoon each of
    - Ground flaxseed
    - Nut butter
- One teaspoon of ground turmeric
- Two teaspoons of maca root powder
- Three-quarter cups of nut milk
- One frozen banana

Method:

1. Blend all the ingredients together to get a smooth mixture.
2. Adjust consistency by adding nut milk.
3. Once done, divide into two glasses and enjoy!

Pituitary Relief Smoothie

Total Prep & Cooking Time: 5 minutes

Yields: 2 servings

Nutrition Facts: Calories: 174 | Carbs: 18.3g | Protein: 9.7g | Fat: 8.3g | Fiber: 14.4g

Ingredients:

- One teaspoon of coconut oil
- One fresh or frozen ripe banana
- One tablespoon of raw sesame seeds
- Two teaspoons each of
  - Chia seeds
  - Raw Maca powder
  - Raw Spirulina
- Two cups of water
- Two tablespoons of hulled hemp seeds

Method:

1. You have to use a blender to process this smoothie. Add the hulled hemp seeds, sesame seeds, and water in the blender and process them. Do it at high speed, and it will only require a minute. This will give you raw-milk like texture.

2. Then, add the following ingredients into it – coconut oil, banana, chia seeds, Maca, and Spirulina, and process the ingredients once again but this time on medium speed for another minute or so. Everything will become well incorporated.

3. You have to drink this smoothie on an empty stomach.

Notes: *In order to make the smoothie rich in antioxidants, you can add some fresh fruits like blueberries, kiwi, and raspberries.*

Chapter 2: Easy Breakfast Recipes

Scrambled Eggs With Feta and Tomatoes

Total Prep & Cooking Time: 10 minutes

Yields: One Plate

Nutrition Facts: Calories: 421 | Carbs: 8.6g | Protein: 20.3g | Fat: 35.1g | Fiber: 1.6g

Ingredients:

- One tbsp. each of
  - Olive oil (extra virgin)
  - Freshly chopped parsley, basil, dill or chives
- Half a cup of cherry tomatoes (each tomato sliced into half)
- Two ounces of crumbled feta cheese (approximately a quarter cup)
- Two eggs are beaten
- Two tbsp. of onion (diced)
- To taste:
  - Black pepper
  - Kosher salt

Method:

1. Keep the beaten eggs in a small-sized bowl and then season it with a pinch of pepper and salt. Set the bowl aside.

2. Use a nonstick skillet to proceed with the cooking. Pour two tbsp. of olive oil. Then add the diced onions. Stir over moderate heat and cook until softened. Make sure that the onions do not look brown. This process should get done by a minute.

3. Add half a cup of tomatoes to skillet and then continue to mix for about two minutes.

4. Now you may add the eggs. Using a spatula, gather the beaten eggs to the center by moving spatula all over the skillet.

5. The eggs will take an additional minute to get cooked. So after that mark, add the parsley or other herbs (if preferred) and feta cheese. Keep the eggs underdone as they will get cooked completely after they are served in the plate itself (from the residual heat). Therefore, cook the entire thing in the skillet for 30 seconds only.

6. Take a serving plate and transfer the eggs to it. Top with some sprinkled parsley and feta cheese, drizzled with some oil, and seasoned with some pepper and salt. These additions are optional and may vary as per your desire.

Smashed Avo and Quinoa

Total Prep & Cooking Time: 15 minutes

Yields: Six bowls

Nutrition Facts: Calories: 492 | Carbs: 67g | Protein: 15g | Fat: 20g | Fiber: 13g

Ingredients:

- One avocado skinned, cut into half, and then pitted
- A handful of cilantro or coriander
- Half a lemon (juiced)
- A quarter red onion (diced finely)
- One-eighth teaspoon of cayenne pepper
- To taste: Sea salt

For the Greens,

- One handful of kale
- One handful of soft herbs (basil, parsley or mint)
- One handful of chard or spinach
- For frying: butter or coconut oil

Serve with,

- One cup of quinoa (cooked)

Method:

1. You will require a frying pan to get this done. To it, add the coconut oil or butter (whichever you prefer) and add the greens. Toss them carefully and then sauté over moderate heat. Stop when they become soft.

2. Mix the onion, cayenne, avocado, cilantro, salt, lemon, and pepper to a bowl and mix them completely. The pepper and salt must be added according to the taste.

3. Add cooked quinoa to the tossed greens and heat altogether over low heat.

4. Take a serving plate and place the quinoa mixture and greens to it. Crown the whole thing with smashed avocado and then serve.

Hormone Balancing Granola

Total Prep & Cooking Time: 35 minutes

Yields: 8 servings

Nutrition Facts: Calories: 360 | Carbs: 19.8g | Protein: 5.1g | Fat: 28.8g | Fiber: 5.8g

Ingredients:

- One-third cup each of

- Flaxseed meal
  - Pumpkin seeds
  - Seedless raisins
- Two teaspoons of cinnamon
- One teaspoon of vanilla extract
- Four tablespoons of maple syrup
- Five tablespoons of melted coconut oil
- A quarter cup of unsweetened coconut flakes
- Two-thirds cup each of
  - Chopped pecans
  - Chopped brazil nuts
- Two tablespoons of ground chia seeds

Method:

1. Set the temperature of the oven to 180 degrees F and preheat.
2. In a food processor, chop the pecans and the Brazil nuts. Then, mix these chopped nuts with coconut flakes, seeds, and other nuts present in the list of ingredients.
3. Add maple syrup, coconut oil, cinnamon, and vanilla extract in a separate bowl and combine well.
4. Now, take the wet ingredients and pour them into the dry ingredients. Mix thoroughly so that everything has become coated properly.
5. Place the prepared mixture in the oven for half an hour and cook.
6. Once done, cut into pieces and serve.

Chapter 3: Healthy Lunch Recipes

Easy Shakshuka

Total Prep & Cooking Time: 30 minutes

Yields: Six servings

Nutrition Facts: Calories: 154 | Carbs: 4.1g | Protein: 9g | Fat: 7.8g | Fiber: 0g

Ingredients:

- Olive oil (extra virgin)
- Two chopped green peppers
- One teaspoon each of
    - Paprika (sweet)
    - Coriander (ground)
- A pinch of red pepper (flakes)
- Half a cup of tomato sauce
- A quarter cup each of
    - Mint leaves (freshly chopped)
    - Parsley leaves (chopped freshly)
- One yellow onion, large-sized (chopped)
- Two cloves of garlic, chopped
- Half a teaspoon of cumin (ground)
- Six cups of chopped tomatoes (Vine-ripe)
- Six large-sized eggs
- To taste: Pepper and salt

Method:

1. You will require a large-sized skillet (made of cast iron). Pour three tablespoons of oil and heat it. After bringing the oil to boil, add the peppers, spices, onions, garlic, pepper, and salt. Stir time to time to cook the veggies for five minutes until they become softened.

2. After the vegetables become soft, add the chopped tomatoes and then tomato sauce. Cover the skillet and simmer for an additional fifteen minutes.

3. Now, you may remove the lid from the pan and then cook a touch more to thicken the consistency. At this point, you may adjust the taste.

4. Make six cavities within the tomato mixture and crack one egg each inside the cavities.

5. Cover the skillet after reducing the heat and allow it to cook so that the eggs settle into the cavities.

6. Keep track of the time and accordingly uncover the skillet and then add mint and parsley. Season with more black and red pepper according to your desire. Serve them warm with the sort of bread you wish.

Ginger Chicken

Total Prep & Cooking Time: 50 minutes

Yields: Six Servings

Nutrition Facts: Calories: 310 | Carbs: 6g | Protein: 37g | Fat: 16g | Fiber: 1g

Ingredients:

- A one-kilogram pack of chicken thighs (skinless and boneless)
- Four cloves of garlic (chopped finely)
- A fifteen-gram pack of coriander (fresh and chopped)
- Two tablespoons of sunflower oil
- One teaspoon each of
    - Turmeric (ground)
    - Chili powder (mild)
- A four hundred milliliter can of coconut milk (reduced-fat)
- One cube of chicken stock
- One ginger properly peeled and chopped finely (it should be of the size of a thumb)
- One lime, juiced
- Two medium-sized onions
- One red chili, sliced and the seeds removed (fresh)

Method:

1. Make the chicken thighs into three large chunks and marinate them with chili powder, garlic, coriander (half of the entire amount), ginger, oil (one tbsp.), and lime juice. Cover the bowl after stirring them well and then store it in the fridge until oven-ready.
2. Marinade the chicken and keep overnight for better flavor.
3. Chop the onions finely (it is going to be the simplest for preparing the curry) before dropping them into the food processor. Pour oil into the frying pan (large-sized) and heat it. Then add chopped onions and stir

them thoroughly for eight minutes until the pieces become soft. Then pour the turmeric powder and stir for an additional minute.

4. Now add the chicken mixture and cook on high heat until you notice a change in its color. Pour the chicken stock, chili, and coconut milk and after covering the pan simmer for another twenty minutes. Sprinkle the left-over coriander leaves and then serve hot.

5. Enjoy.

Carrot and Miso Soup

Total Prep & Cooking Time: 1 hour

Yields: Four bowls of soup

Nutrition Facts: Calories: 76 | Carbs: 8.76g | Protein: 4.83g | Fat: 2.44g | Fiber: 1.5g

Ingredients:

- Two tbsps. of oil
- Garlic, minced (four cloves)
- One inch of garlic (grated)
- Three tbsps. of miso paste (white)
- One diced onion
- One pound of carrot (sliced thinly)
- Four cups of vegetable stock
- To taste: Pepper and Salt

For garnishing,

- Two scallions (sliced thinly)
- Chili pepper (seven spices)
- One nori roasted (make thin slivers)
- Sesame oil

Method:

1. Using a soup pot will be convenient to proceed with. Pour oil in a pot and then heat over a high flame. Now you may put garlic, carrot, and onion and sauté them thoroughly. Cook for about ten minutes so that the onions turn translucent.

2. Then add the ginger and vegetable stock. Mix them well and cook all together. Put the flame to simmer. Cover the pot while cooking to make the carrot tender. This will take another thirty minutes.

3. Put off the flame and puree the soup with the help of an immersion blender.

4. Use a small-sized bowl to whisk together a spoonful of the soup and the white miso paste. Stir until the paste dissolve and pour the mixture back to the pot.

5. Add pepper and salt if required.

6. Divide the soup among four bowls and enrich its feel by adding scallions, sesame oil, seven spices, and nori.

Arugula Salad

Total Prep & Cooking Time: 1 hour 10 minutes

Yields: Two bowls of salad

Nutrition Facts: Calories: 336.8 | Carbs: 30.6g | Protein: 7.7g | Fat: 22.2g | Fiber: 7.3g

Ingredients:

For the salad,

- Two medium-sized beets (boiled or roasted for about an hour), skinned and sliced into pieces that can easily be bitten
- Four tablespoons of goat cheese
- Approximately 2.5 oz. of baby arugula (fresh)
- A quarter cup of walnuts (chopped roughly before toasting)

For the dressing,

- Three tablespoons of olive oil (extra virgin)
- A quarter tsp. each of
  - Mustard powder (dried)
  - Pepper
- Half a tsp. each of
  - Salt
  - Sugar

- One and a half tablespoons of lemon juice

Method:

1. For preparing the vinaigrette, place all the ingredients (listed in the dressing ingredients section) in a jar and then shake them to emulsify. At this stage, before starting with the process of emulsification, you may add or remove the ingredients as per your liking.

2. Get the salad assembled (again depending upon the taste you want to give it), add a fistful of arugula leaves, place some chopped beets (after they have been cooked), and finally the toasted walnuts (already chopped).

3. Drizzle vinaigrette over the salad and enjoy.

Notes:

- *Coat the beets with oil (olive), roll them up in an aluminum foil, and then roast the beets at a temperature of 400 degrees F.*

- *And for boiling the beets, immerse them in water after transferring to a pot and simmer them for 45 minutes.*

Kale Soup

Total Prep & Cooking Time: 55 minutes

Yields: 8 servings

Nutrition Facts: Calories: 277.3 | Carbs: 50.9g | Protein: 9.6g | Fat: 4.5g | Fiber: 10.3g

Ingredients:

- Two tbsps. of dried parsley
- One tbsp. of Italian seasoning
- Salt and pepper
- Thirty oz. of drained cannellini beans
- Six peeled and cubed white potatoes
- Fifteen ounces of diced tomatoes
- Six vegetable Bouillon cubes
- Eight cups of water
- One bunch of kale (with chopped leaves and stems removed)
- Two tbsps. of chopped garlic
- One chopped yellow onion
- Two tbsps. of olive oil

Method:

1. At first, take a large soup pot, add in some olive oil, and heat it.
2. Add garlic and onion. Cook them until soft.
3. Then stir in the kale and cook for about two minutes, until wilted.
4. Pour the water and add the beans, potatoes, tomatoes, vegetable bouillon, parsley, and the Italian seasoning.
5. On medium heat, simmer the soup for about twenty-five minutes, until the potatoes are cooked through.
6. Finally, do the seasoning with salt and pepper according to your taste.

Roasted Sardines

Total Prep & Cooking Time: 25 minutes

Yields: 4 servings

Nutrition Facts: Calories: 418 | Carbs: 2.6g | Protein: 41g | Fat: 27.2g | Fiber: 0.8g

Ingredients:

- 3.5 oz. of cherry tomatoes (cut them in halves)
- One medium-sized red onion (chopped finely)
- Two tablespoons each of
    - Chopped parsley
    - Extra-virgin olive oil
- One clove of garlic (halved)
- Eight units of fresh sardines (gutted and cleaned, heads should be cleaned)
- A quarter teaspoon of chili flakes
- One teaspoon of toasted cumin seeds
- Half a lemon (zested and juiced)

Method:

1. Set the temperature of the oven to 180 degrees C and preheat. Take a roasting tray and grease it lightly.

2. Take a bowl and add the tomatoes and onions in it. Add the lemon juice too and toss the veggies in the lemon juice. Now, add the zest, olive oil, chili, cumin, garlic, and parsley and toss everything once again.

3. Use pepper and salt to season the mixture. The cavity of the sardines has to be filled. Use some of the tomato and onion mixture for this purpose. Once done, place the sardines on the prepared roasting tray. Take the remaining mixture and scatter it over the sardines.

4. Roast the sardines for about 10-15 minutes, and by the end of this, they should be cooked thoroughly.

5. Serve and enjoy!

Chapter 4: Tasty Dinner Recipes

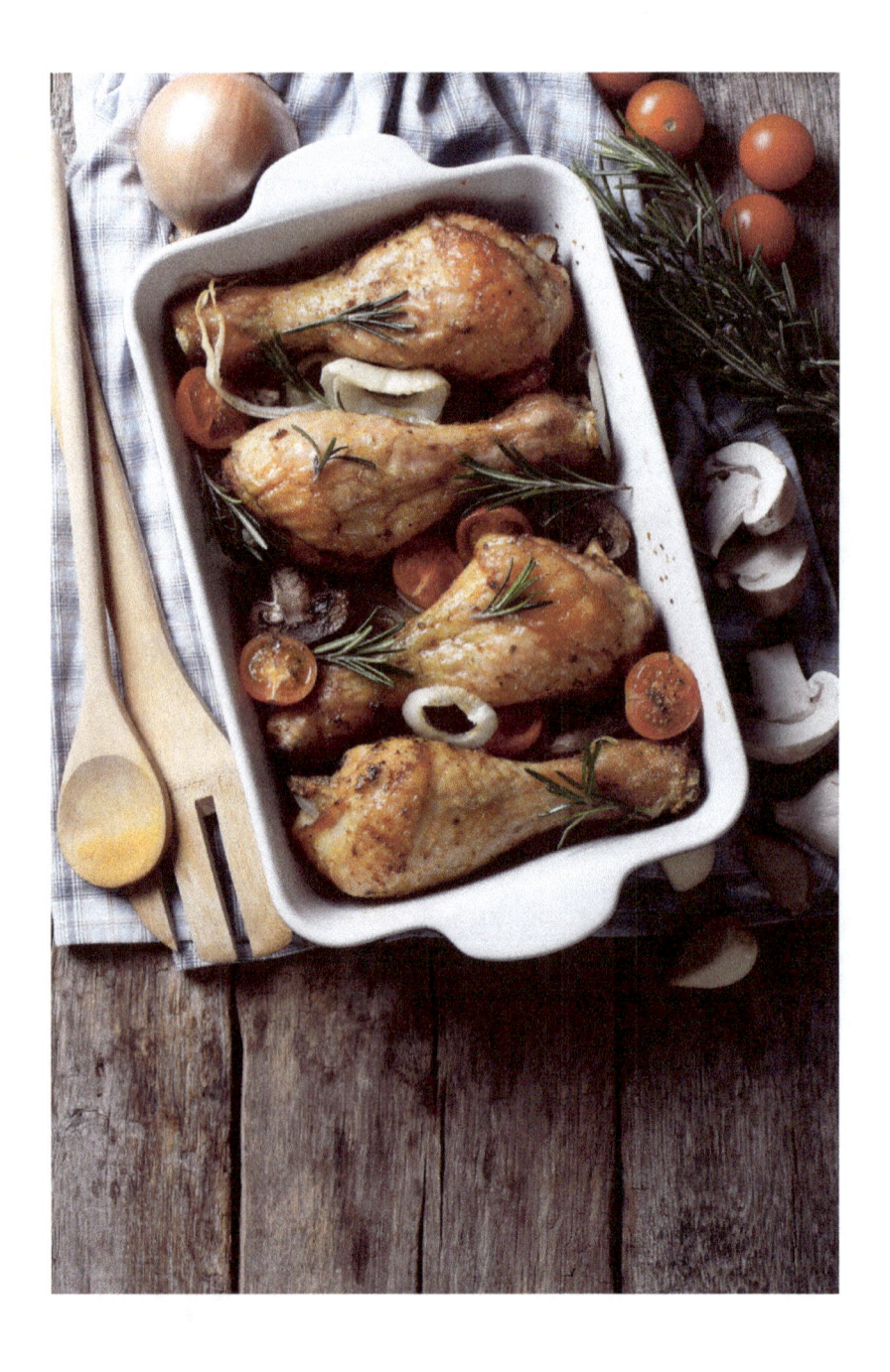

Rosemary Chicken

Total Prep & Cooking Time: 50 minutes

Yields: 4 servings

Nutrition Facts: Calories: 232 | Carbs: 3.9g | Protein: 26.7g | Fat: 11.6g | Fiber: 0.3g

Ingredients:

- Four chicken breast halves (skinless and boneless)
- One-eighth tsp. kosher salt
- One-fourth tsp. ground black pepper
- One and a half tbsps. of lemon juice
- One and a half tbsps. of Dijon mustard
- Two tbsps. of freshly minced rosemary
- Three tbsps. of olive oil
- Eight minced garlic cloves

Method:

1. At first, preheat a grill to medium-high heat. The grate needs to be lightly oiled.
2. Take a bowl and add lemon juice, mustard, rosemary, olive oil, garlic, salt, and ground black pepper. Whisk them together.
3. Take a resealable plastic bag and place the chicken breasts in it. Over the chicken, pour the garlic mixture (reserve one-eighth cup of it).
4. Seal the bag and start massaging the marinade gently into the chicken. Allow it to stand for about thirty minutes at room temperature.
5. Then on the preheated grill, place the chicken and cook for about four minutes.
6. Flip the chicken and baste it with the marinade reserved and then cook for about five minutes, until thoroughly cooked.

Finally, cover it with a foil and allow it to rest for about 2 minutes before you serve them.

Corned Beef and Cabbage

Total Prep & Cooking Time: 2 hours 35 minutes

Yields: 5 servings

Nutrition Facts: Calories: 868.8 | Carbs: 75.8g | Protein: 50.2g | Fat: 41.5g | Fiber: 14g

Ingredients:

- One big cabbage head (cut it into small wedges)
- Five peeled carrots (chopped into three-inch pieces)
- Ten red potatoes (small)
- Three pounds of corned beef brisket (along with the packet of spice)

Method:

1. At first, in a Dutch oven or a large pot, place the corned beef, and cover it with water. Then add in the spices from the packet of spices that came along with the beef. Cover the pot, bring it to a boil, and finally reduce it to a simmer. Allow it to simmer for about 2 hours and 30 minutes or until tender.

2. Add carrots and whole potatoes, and cook them until the vegetables are tender. Add the cabbage wedges and cook for another fifteen minutes. Then finally remove the meat and allow it to rest for fifteen minutes.

3. Take a bowl, place the vegetables in it, and cover it. Add broth (which is reserved in the pot) as much as you want. Then finally cut the meat against the grain.

Roasted Parsnips and Carrots

Total Prep & Cooking Time: 1 hour

Yields: 4 servings

Nutrition Facts: Calories: 112 | Carbs: 27g | Protein: 2g | Fat: 1g | Fiber: 7g

Ingredients:

- Two tbsps. of freshly minced parsley or dill
- One and a half tsp. of freshly ground black pepper
- One tbsp. kosher salt
- Three tbsps. of olive oil
- One pound of unpeeled carrots
- Two pounds of peeled parsnips

Method:

1. At first, preheat your oven to 425 degrees.
2. If the carrots and parsnips are thick, then cut them into halves lengthwise.
3. Then, slice each of them diagonally into one inch thick slices. Don't cut them too small because the vegetables will anyway shrink while you cook them.
4. Take a sheet pan, and place the cut vegetables on it.
5. Then add some olive oil, pepper, salt, and toss them nicely.
6. Roast them for about twenty to forty minutes (the roasting time depends on the size of the vegetables), accompanied by occasional tossing. Continue to roast until the carrots and parsnips become tender.
7. Finally, sprinkle some dill and serve.

Herbed Salmon

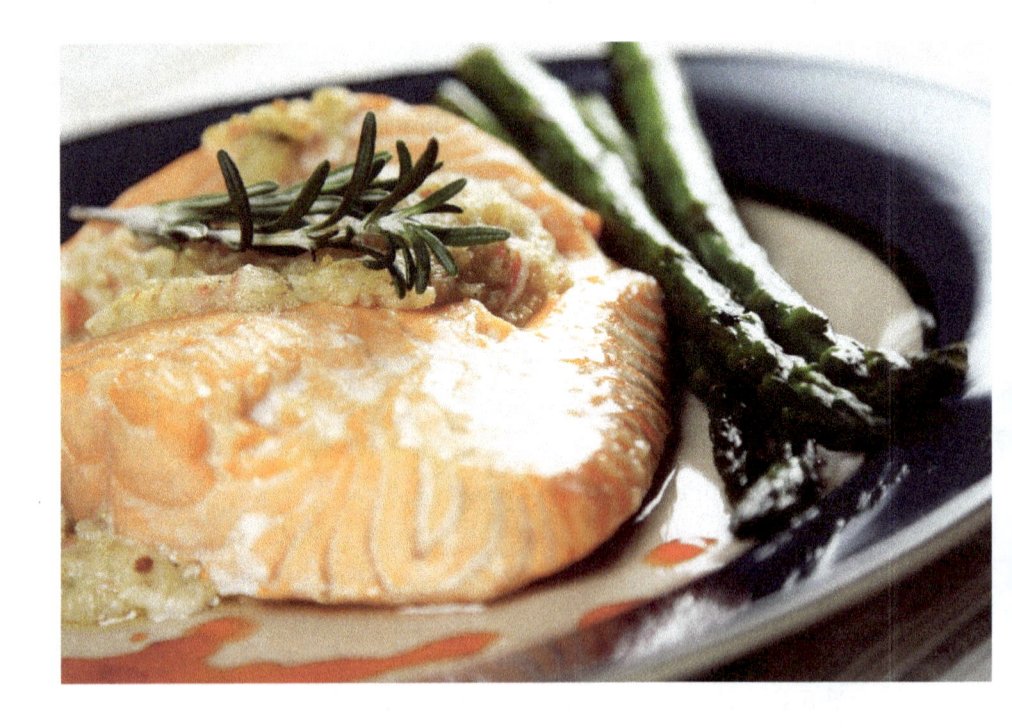

Total Prep & Cooking Time: 30 minutes

Yields: 4 servings

Nutrition Facts: Calories: 301 | Carbs: 1g | Protein: 29g | Fat: 19g | Fiber: 0g

Ingredients:

- Half a tsp. of dried thyme or two tsps. of freshly minced thyme
- Half a tsp. of pepper

- Three-fourth tsp. of salt
- One tbsp. of olive oil
- One tbsp. freshly minced rosemary or one tsp. of crushed dried rosemary.
- Four minced cloves of garlic
- Four (six ounces) fillets of salmon

Method:

1. At first, preheat your oven to 425 degrees.
2. Take a 15 by 10 by 1 inch baking pan and grease it.
3. Place the salmon on it while keeping the skin side down.
4. Combine the garlic cloves, rosemary, thyme, salt, and pepper. Spread it evenly over the salmon fillets.
5. Roast them for about fifteen to eighteen minutes until they reach your desired doneness.

Chipotle Cauliflower Tacos

Total Prep & Cooking Time: 30 minutes

Yields: 8 servings

Nutrition Facts: Calories: 440 | Carbs: 51.6g | Protein: 10.1g | Fat: 24g | Fiber: 9g

Ingredients:

For the tacos,

- Four tablespoons of avocado oil
- One head of cauliflower (large-sized, chopped into bite-sized florets)
- One cup of cilantro (freshly chopped)
- One tablespoon each of
    - Fresh lime juice
    - Maple syrup or honey
- Two tsps. of chipotle adobo sauce
- Cracked black pepper
- One teaspoon of salt
- 4-8 units of garlic cloves (freshly minced)

For the Chipotle Aioli,

- A quarter cup of chipotle adobo sauce
- Half a cup each of
    - Sour cream
    - Clean mayo

One teaspoon of sea salt

Two cloves of garlic (minced)

For serving,

- Almond flour tortillas
- Guacamole
- Almond ricotta cheese
- Sliced tomatoes, radish, and cabbage

Method:

1. Set the temperature of the oven to 425 degrees F. Now, use parchment paper to line a pan. Take the bite-sized florets of the cauliflower and spread them evenly on the pan. Use 2-4 tbsps. of avocado oil, pepper, salt, and minced garlic and drizzle it on the pan.

2. Roast the cauliflower for half an hour at 425 degrees F and halfway through the process, flip the florets.

3. When you are roasting the cauliflower, take the rest of the ingredients of the cauliflower and mix them in a bowl. Once everything has been properly incorporated, set the mixture aside.

4. Now, take another bowl and in it, add the ingredients of the chipotle aioli. Mix them and set the bowl aside.

5. If you have any other taco fixings, get them ready.

6. Once the cauliflower is ready, toss the florets in the chipotle sauce.

7. Serve the cauliflower in tortillas along with fixings of your choice and the chipotle aioli.

PART III

Chapter 1: Tasty Breakfast Options

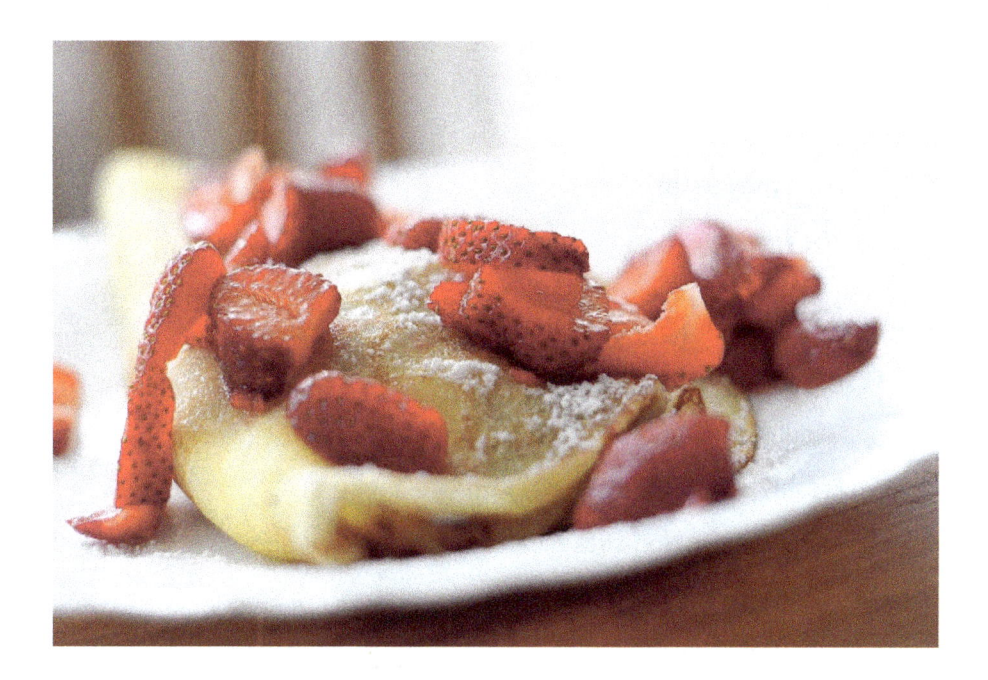

French Crepe

Servings Provided: 8

Time Required: 20 minutes

What is Needed:

The Crepes:

- Eggs (2)
- Melted butter (.25 cup)
- Sugar (2.5 tbsp.)

- A-P flour (.5 cup)
- Milk (.5 cup)
- Water (.125 cup)
- Vanilla (.5 tsp.)
- Dash (tiny dash)

The Filling:

- Powdered sugar (2-4 tbsp./as desired)
- Heavy whipping cream (1 cup)
- Vanilla extract (.5 tsp.)
- Freshly sliced strawberries
- Also Needed: Non-stick - 6-inch skillet

Preparation Method:

1. Prepare the crepes. Whisk all the fixings except the flour.
2. Fold in the flour - a little bit at a time - whisking just until the flour is incorporated.
3. Let the crepe batter rest for ten minutes. Whisk again before using it.
4. Grease the skillet with unsalted butter and warm it using the medium-temperature setting.
5. Pour about two to three tablespoons of batter into the pan - while tipping the pan from side to side to get the mixture spreading over the pan.
6. Cook each side of the crepe for half a minute before gently loosening the edges with a large spatula. If it lifts, it's ready to be

flipped. If not, cook it for another 10-15 seconds and try again. Gently lift the crepe out of the pan, then flip over into the pan and cook the other side for another 10-15 seconds; remove to cool.
7. Prepare the filling. Use a hand/stand mixer to beat the heavy whipping cream until soft peaks form. Add in the powdered sugar and vanilla. Continue mixing until stiff peaks form.
8. Spread a layer of cream over each crepe, sliced strawberries, and roll the crepe as you would a wrap.

French Omelette

Servings Provided: 1

Time Required: 15 minutes

What is Needed:

- Milk (1 tbsp.)
- Egg (1)
- Basil (1 tbsp.)
- Chives (1 tbsp.)
- Tarragon (.5 tbsp.)
- Salt and pepper (a pinch of each)
- Olive oil (as needed for the pan)
- Sundried tomato (1 thinly sliced - oil drained)
- Crumbled goat cheese (1 tbsp.)

Preparation Method:

1. Chop the basil, tarragon, and chives.
2. Whisk the milk, egg, salt, and pepper in a small mixing container. Add half of the fresh herbs and gently stir to combine.
3. Add one tablespoon of olive oil to a small pan. Warm the oil using medium heat as you swirl it around the pan so that it coats the entire bottom of the pan and a little bit along the sides of the pan.
4. Dump the egg mixture into the pan. Swirl the pan so that the egg batter goes to the edges of the pan. Use a rubber spatula to gently push the egg batter to the edges of the pan.
5. Once the egg batter looks set on the bottom and is starting to bubble up a bit, lift the pan while tilting it to one side to slide the egg onto an awaiting using a large spatula. Flip the egg onto its other side into the pan and place it back on the burner using low heat.
6. Toss the crumbled cheese and tomato slices into the center of the omelet. Gently fold one side of the egg over, folding one more time - over itself (into thirds).
7. Serve promptly, garnished with the remaining fresh herbs.

Chapter 2: Delicious Salads

Traditional French Country Salad With Lemon Dijon **Vinaigrette**

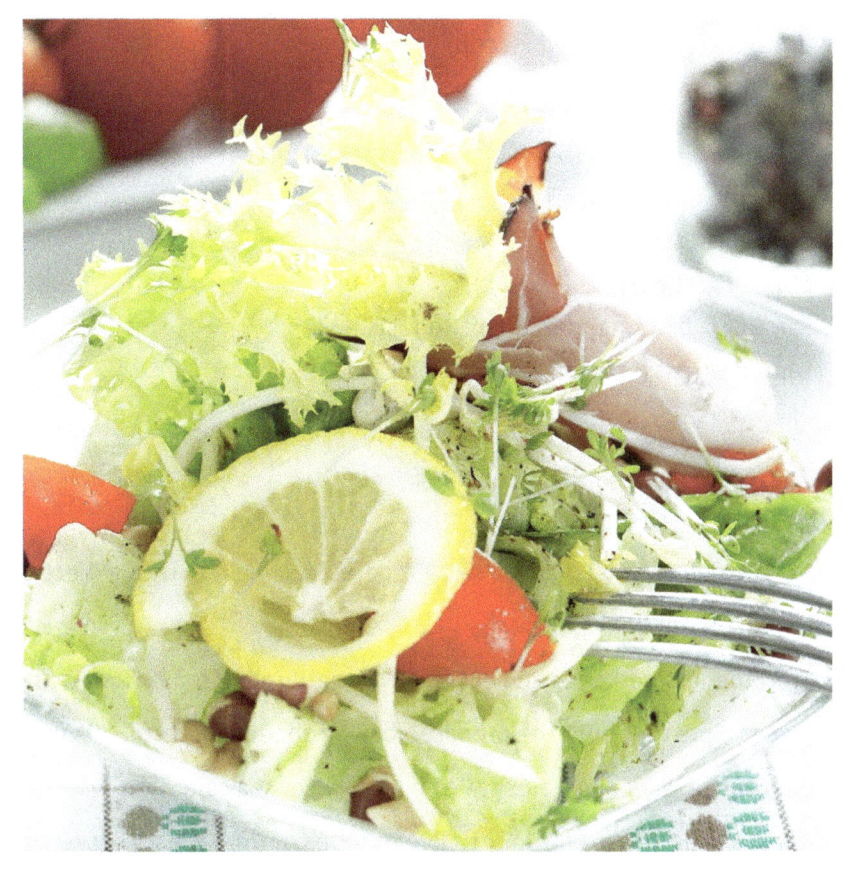

Servings Provided: 4

Time Required: 20 minutes

What is Needed:

- Arugula (5 oz. bag)
- Asparagus (.5 lb.)
- Olive oil (as desired)
- Sea salt (as desired)
- Sliced cooked beets (.5 cup)
- Whole walnuts or pecans, toasted (.5 cup)
- Crumbled goat cheese (.25 cup)

The Vinaigrette:

- Balsamic vinegar (3 tbsp.)
- Dijon mustard (2 tbsp.)
- Olive oil (2 tbsp.)
- Minced garlic cloves (2 small)
- Sea salt & black pepper(.5 tsp./to taste)
- Lemon & zest (half of 1 lemon)

Preparation Method:

1. Set the oven at 400° Fahrenheit. Prepare a baking tray with a piece of parchment baking paper.
2. Trim the tattered ends and cut the asparagus into 1.5-inch long pieces. Spread it onto the prepared baking sheet. Drizzle the olive oil over the asparagus along with a sprinkle of sea salt.
3. Roast the asparagus for four to five minutes or until the asparagus is tender but still has a bite. Let it cool.
4. Toss the arugula with the asparagus in a large bowl.
5. Prepare the dressing. Whisk all of the vinaigrette fixings in a small measuring cup.
6. Assemble the salad. Toss the salad with the vinaigrette until

everything is lightly coated, and garnish it using sliced beets, toasted nuts, and crumbled goat cheese.

Chapter 3: Soup

Classic French Onion Bistro Soup

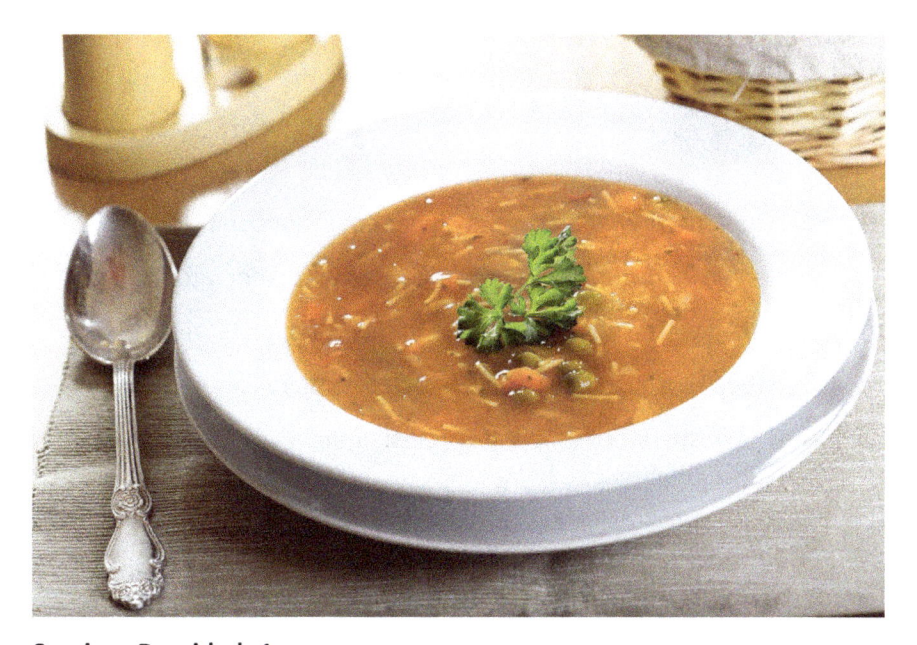

Servings Provided: 4

Time Required: 1.5 hours

What is Needed:

- Onions, (8 cups sliced/2 extra-large)
- Unsalted butter (1.5 tbsp.)
- Oil (1 tbsp.)
- Salt (.5 tsp.)
- Sugar (1 pinch)

- A-P flour (1.5 tbsp.)
- Low-sodium beef broth (4 cups)
- Pepper & salt (as desired)
- Sliced crusty French bread
- Gruyere cheese for the top/gruyere-cheddar mix (4 oz.)
- Also Needed: Oven-proof bowls (4)

Preparation Method:

1. Melt the butter with oil over low heat in a large pot or dutch oven. Slice the onions into crescent shapes and toss them into the pan. Place a lid on the pan and simmer them for about 15 minutes.
2. Slice the bread into ½-inch slices and toast them (set aside).
3. Adjust the stovetop temperature setting slightly higher and stir in the salt and sugar. Simmer with the lid off for another 40 to 45 minutes until onions have caramelized. Stir them occasionally throughout the duration.
4. Sprinkle the flour into the pot, stir, and simmer an additional three minutes.
5. Slowly add the broth into the pot, stirring as your pour. Season with a pinch of salt and pepper and cook for another 20 minutes until simmering and hot.
6. Warm the oven at 350° Fahrenheit.
7. Once the soup is ready, divide the soup into bowls. Place four to five baguette slices into each bowl. Top each bowl with grated cheese (.25 cup each dish).
8. Bake them until the cheese completely melts and serve promptly.

Fresh French Pea Soup

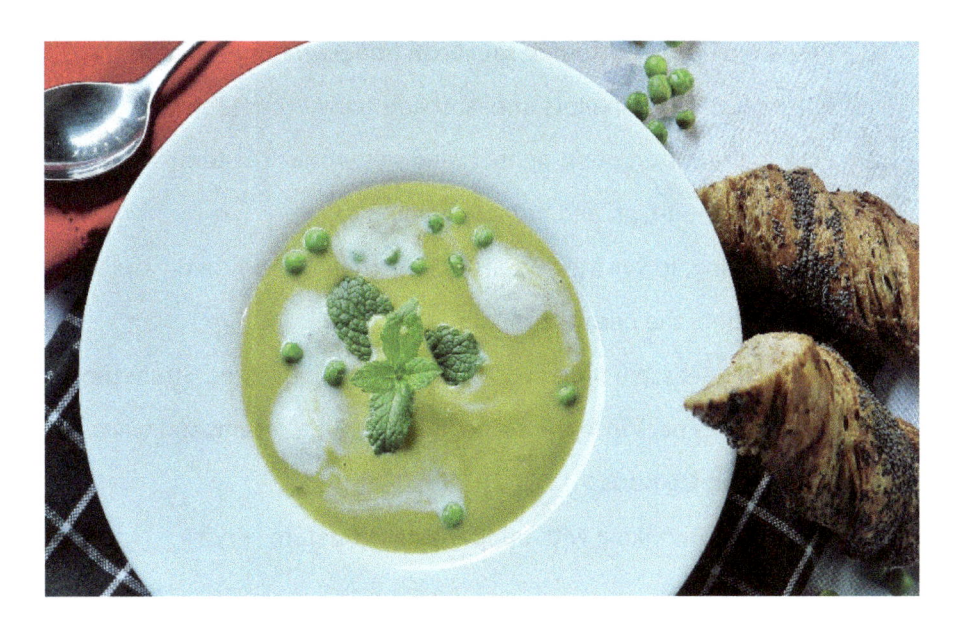

Servings Provided: 4

Time Required: 17 minutes

What is Needed:

- Butter with salt (2 tbsp.)
- Shallots (2 medium)
- Water (2 cups)
- Fresh green peas (3 cups)
- Table salt (.25 tsp.)
- Heavy whipping cream (3 tbsp.)

Preparation Method:

1. Prepare a heavy-bottomed saucepan (medium temp) to melt the butter. Sauté the shallots until soft and translucent (3 min.).
2. Pour in the water, peas, pepper, and salt. Adjust the temperature setting to med-high and bring to a boil.
3. Once boiling, lower the temperature setting to low, cover, and simmer until the peas are tender (12-18 min.).
4. Puree the peas in a food processor/blender in batches. Strain the pureed peas back into the saucepan, stir in the cream, and warm until it's piping hot.
5. Season to your liking with pepper and salt before serving.

Green Vegetable Soup

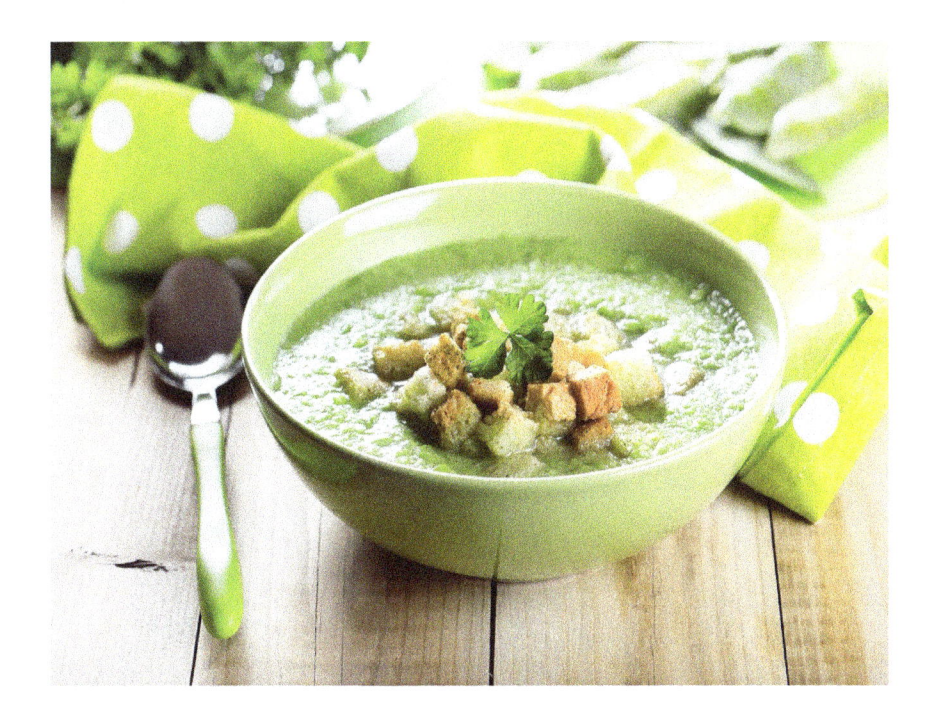

Servings Provided: 6

Time Required: 1 hour 40 minutes

What is Needed:

- Onions (2)
- Garlic (3 cloves)
- Butter, with salt (3 tbsp.)
- Swanson Clear Chicken Broth CAM (2 - 14.5 oz. cans)
- Water (4.5 cups)

- Carrots (3)
- Leeks (1)
- Spring onions/scallions - include tops & bulb (3)
- Habanero pepper (1 ½)
- Spinach (10 oz. bag)
- Watercress (1 bunch - raw)
- Table salt (1 tbsp.)
- Extra-virgin olive oil NOI (.25 cup)
- Red wine vinegar (50 Grain) NAK (.125 cup)

Preparation Method:

1. Warm a skillet using the med-high temperature setting. Sauté the minced garlic and onion (5 min.).
2. Add the water, chicken stock, spinach, carrots, green onions, leeks, habanero peppers, and watercress. Prepare it using a low-boil until the carrots are softened (30 min.). Remove the pan from the burner, and cool it for about half an hour.
3. When cooled, puree the soup in a food processor until smooth. Pour the mixture into the pot, and simmer using the low-temperature setting for 15 minutes.
4. Serve with a drizzle of olive oil and vinegar to your liking.

Chapter 4: Beef Options

Beef Bourguignon - Slow-Cooked

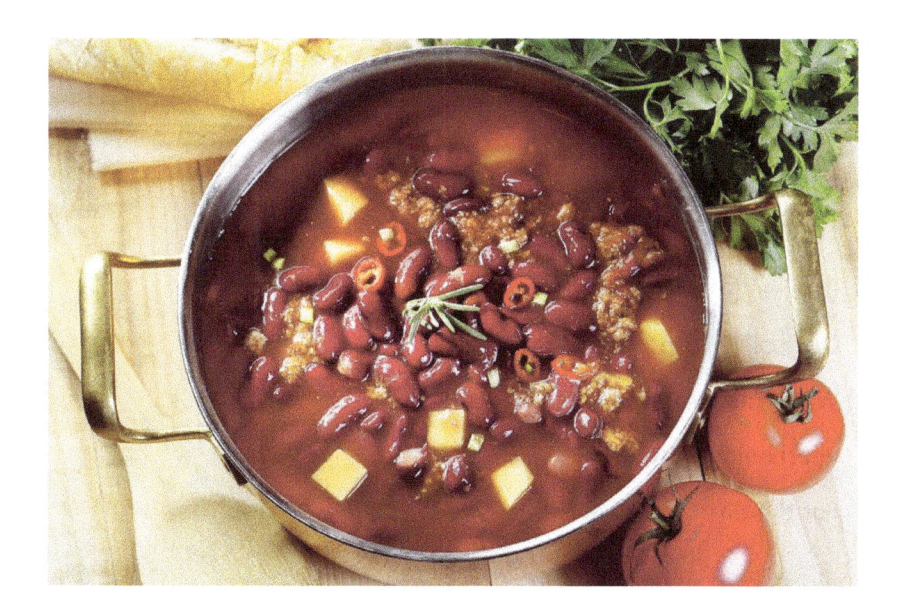

Servings Provided: 6

Time Required: 2.5 hours

What is Needed:

- Bacon (6 oz. - diced)
- Beef chuck (3 lb.)
- Large onion (1 chopped)

- Carrots (1)
- Garlic (2 minced cloves)
- A-P flour (3 tbsp.)
- Beef broth (1.5 cups)
- Red wine (¼ of a bottle)
- Salt (1 tsp.)
- Black pepper (1 pinch)
- Rosemary (1 sprig)
- Thyme (2 sprigs)
- Bay leaf (1)
- Olive oil (2 tbsp.)
- White mushrooms (7-8 thick slices)
- Pearl onions (10 oz.)
- For the Garnish: Fresh parsley

Preparation Method:

1. Warm a dutch oven or other large pot to cook the diced bacon using the med-high temperature setting. When it's nicely browned, transfer it to a paper-lined platter using a slotted spoon. Save the diced bacon for breakfast or a dish of mashed potatoes or just trash it.
2. Slice the beef into two-inch portions and toss it into the pot to brown each side. Remove the meat from the pan.
3. Chop and mix in the onion to sauté until it's translucent (5 min.). Mince and add the garlic to sauté for about half a minute.

4. Add the beef back into the pot and dust it with three tablespoons of flour. Stir the meat until the flour has been absorbed (1 min.).
5. Add in the beef broth and just enough red wine to almost fully immerse it in juices. Stir and add a teaspoon of pepper and salt as desired.
6. Tie the rosemary, thyme, and bay leaf together with a piece of kitchen twine, and drop the bouquet into the pot. Slice the carrots in half lengthwise, then cut into one-inch wide pieces, and add the carrots into the pot as well. Simmer them using the medium temperature setting. Cover the pot with a lid and adjust the temperature setting to med-low. Simmer the stew for about 2.2 to 3 hours until the beef is very tender.
7. Warm the olive oil in a large skillet using the med-low temperature setting. Add the sliced mushrooms and pearl onions, cooking until both are softened (7-8 min.). Set aside until ready to serve.
8. After the beef is ready, remove the herb packet.
9. Prepare a shallow bowl with the meat, sautéed mushrooms, pearl onions, and carrots. Add the sauce and garnish with a portion of chopped parsley.

Entrecote Steak With Red Wine Sauce

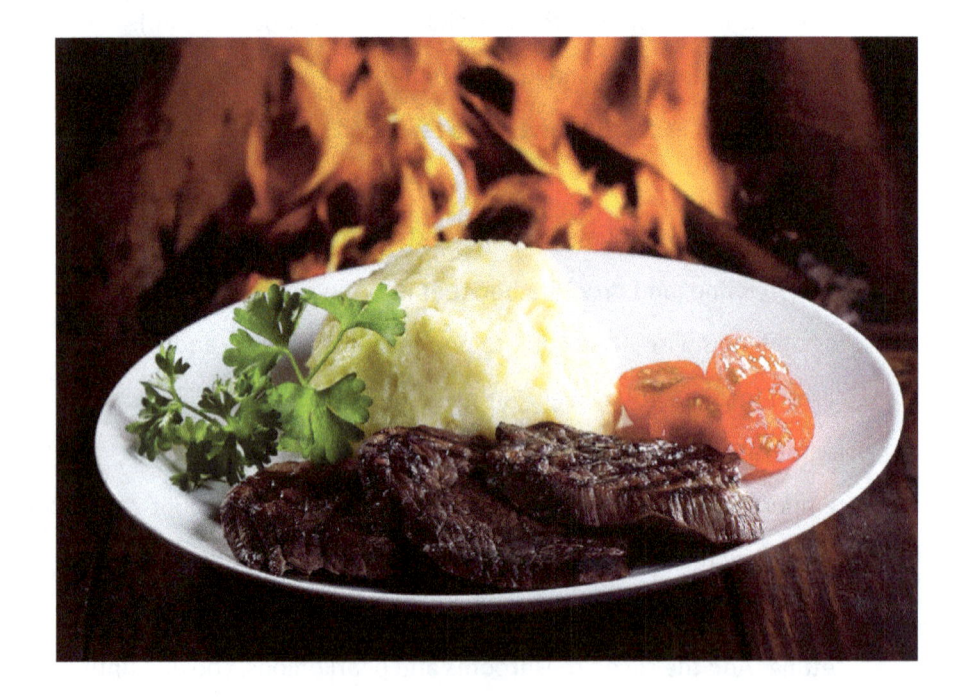

Servings Provided: 2

Time Required: 16 minutes

What is Needed:

- Rib-eye steaks (2 small)
- Black pepper & salt (as desired)
- Butter - unsalted (3 tbsp.)
- Shallot (1)
- Red wine (3 tbsp.)

- Beef stock (1/3 cup + 1 tbsp.)
- To Garnish: freshly chopped parsley

Preparation Method:

1. Generously sprinkle the steaks with pepper and salt.
2. Warm a cast-iron skillet using the high-temperature setting until it's 'smoking' hot. Add 1.5 tablespoons of butter to the pan, adjusting the setting to med-high.
3. Add the steaks to the hot buttered pan to cook for three minutes per side (medium doneness). Transfer the steaks to a platter for now.
4. Finely chop and add the shallot to the pan and sauté them for about a minute. Add the wine, and scrape the tasty browned bits with the juices from the bottom of the pan.
5. Reduce the temperature setting to medium, and stir in the beef stock. Simmer the mixture until the liquid has reduced by about half. Stir in the rest of the butter and prepare to serve it.
6. Use a sharp knife to slice the steaks at an angle and add the sauce. Garnish with a portion of fresh parsley.
7. Serve with your favorite side dish (ex. mashed potatoes, veggies, or french fries).

Pan-Seared Steak au Poivre

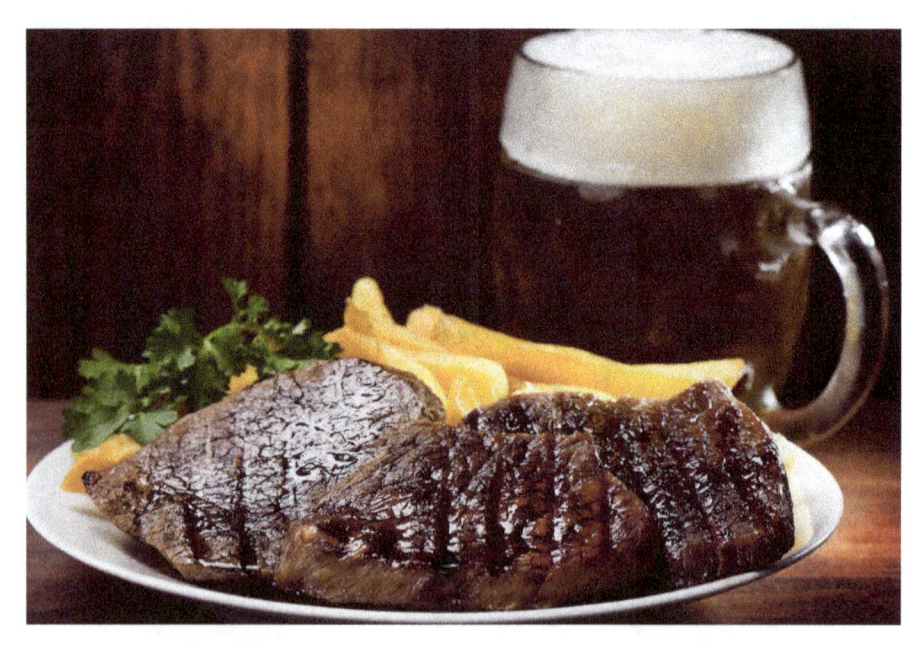

Servings Provided: 4

Time Required: 30 minutes

What is Needed:

- Filet mignons (4 small 1-inch each)
- Black peppercorns - cracked (1 tbsp.)
- Beef broth (.5 cup)
- Olive oil (1 tbsp.)
- Optional: Cognac (.25 cup)
- Cubed butter (2 tbsp.)

Preparation Method:

1. Use a paper towel to pat dry each filet and dust with pepper.
2. Warm a heavy cast-iron skillet using the medium-high heat until it's 'smoking' hot.
3. Flip the steaks and cook until small drops of red juice come to the surface (5 min. for medium). Transfer to a platter and keep them warm until time to add them to the mixture.
4. Empty the broth into the skillet to heat using the high-temperature setting and scrape up any browned bits.
5. At this point, add in the cognac and boil for one to two minutes to burn off the alcohol.
6. Remove the skillet from the burner. Whisk in the butter one cube at a time until melted.
7. Pour the sauce over the steaks and serve.

Steak Diane

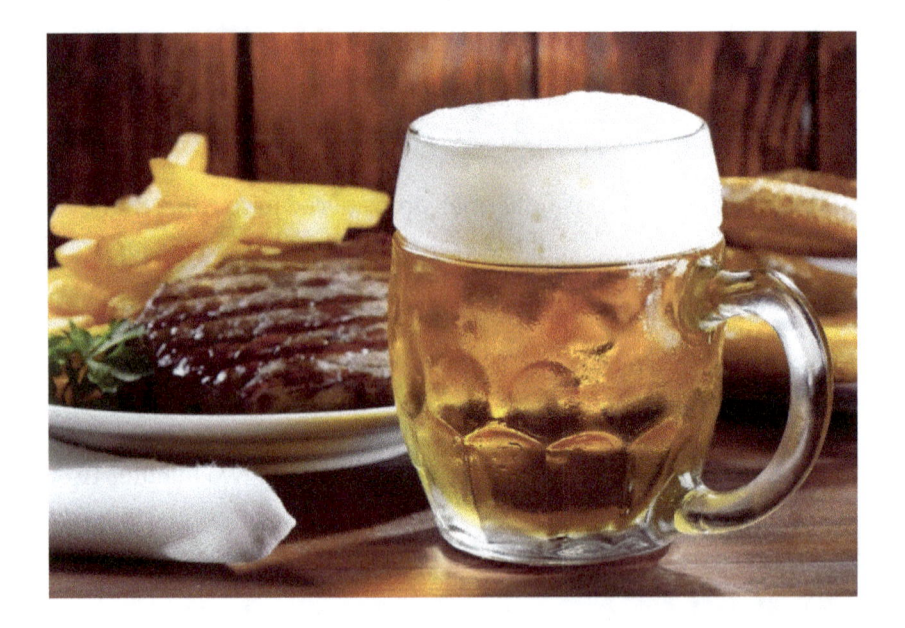

Servings Provided: 2

Time Required: 30 minutes

What is Needed:

- Jus De Veau Lie/Veal Demi-Glace-Pwd FD (.5 cup)
- Dijon Mustard NB (1 tbsp.)
- Worcestershire Sauce (2 tsp.)
- Tomato paste - salt added (1 tsp. - canned)
- Spices - pepper, red or cayenne (1 pinch)

    The Steaks:

- Soybean oil (2 tsp.)
- Beef tenderloin (2 - 8 oz. trimmed to ¼- inch thickness)
- Black pepper & kosher salt (as desired)
- Butter - no-salt (1 tbsp.)
- Shallots (3 tbsp.)
- Cognac (.25 cup)
- Heavy whipping cream (.25 cup)
- Chives (2 tsp.)

Preparation Method:

1. Generously sprinkle the steaks with salt. Wait for them to reach room temperature while you make the sauce.
2. Use the high-temperature setting to warm the oil. Once it reaches a smoking point, add the steaks, and dot them with a few chunks of butter.
3. Sear the meat (high temp) until brown on each side, two to three minutes on each side, keeping them on the rare side (internal temp of 125° Fahrenheit. Transfer steaks to a warm plate.
4. Toss the shallots into the skillet and sauté them until softened (2-3 min.).
5. Remove the skillet to a cool burner and add in the Cognac. Carefully ignite it using a fireplace lighter. After the alcohol burns off and the flames go out, return the skillet to the high setting and wait for it to boil. Simmer for a few minutes to reduce its volume slightly.
6. Add demi-glace mixture, cream, and any accumulated juices from

the steak. Cook on high heat just until the sauce starts to thicken (3-5 min.).
7. Transfer the steaks back into the pan and adjust the temperature setting to low. Gently simmer until meat is heated through and cooked to your desired level of doneness.
8. Serve on a heated plate with a generous portion of sauce. Sprinkle with chives to your liking and serve.

Chapter 5: Other Delicious French Classics

French Ham & Grilled Cheese Sandwich - Croque Monsieur

Servings Provided: 4

Time Required: 25 minutes

What is Needed:

- Sourdough toast (8 slices)
- Gruyere cheese (8 oz.)
- Black forest ham (8 slices)
- Bechamel sauce (1 recipe)
- Dijon mustard

    The Sauce:

- Whole milk (1 cup)

- Unsalted butter (1 tbsp.)
- A-P flour (2 tbsp.)
- Pepper and salt (to your liking)

Preparation Method:

1. Make the sauce by warming the milk in a small saucepan using the med-low temperature setting until steam rises from the milk, but it has yet to boil. *Don't boil.*
2. Use another saucepan to melt the butter. Sift in the flour to create a bubbly, paste-like mixture. Slowly pour in hot milk, whisking it with a pinch of salt and pepper to your liking.
3. Stir the bechamel sauce using the low-temperature setting until it's thick enough to coat the back of a wooden spoon.
4. Set the oven using the broil function. Toast the bread slices and spread them with the mustard over half of the bread.
5. Prepare the sandwich using two slices of ham and shredded cheese on each. Top it using the ham with more shredded cheese.
6. Put the remaining bread slices over the ham and cheese to assemble the sandwiches. Spread about one to two tablespoons of bechamel sauce over the top of each sandwich. Sprinkle more shredded cheese on top of the bechamel.
7. Place the sandwiches on a baking tray and place the pan on the center oven rack until the cheese starts to melt.
8. Move the sandwiches to the top rack for about 30 seconds, removing when the cheese starts to obtain little golden spots.

Pork Chops With Mustard Sauce

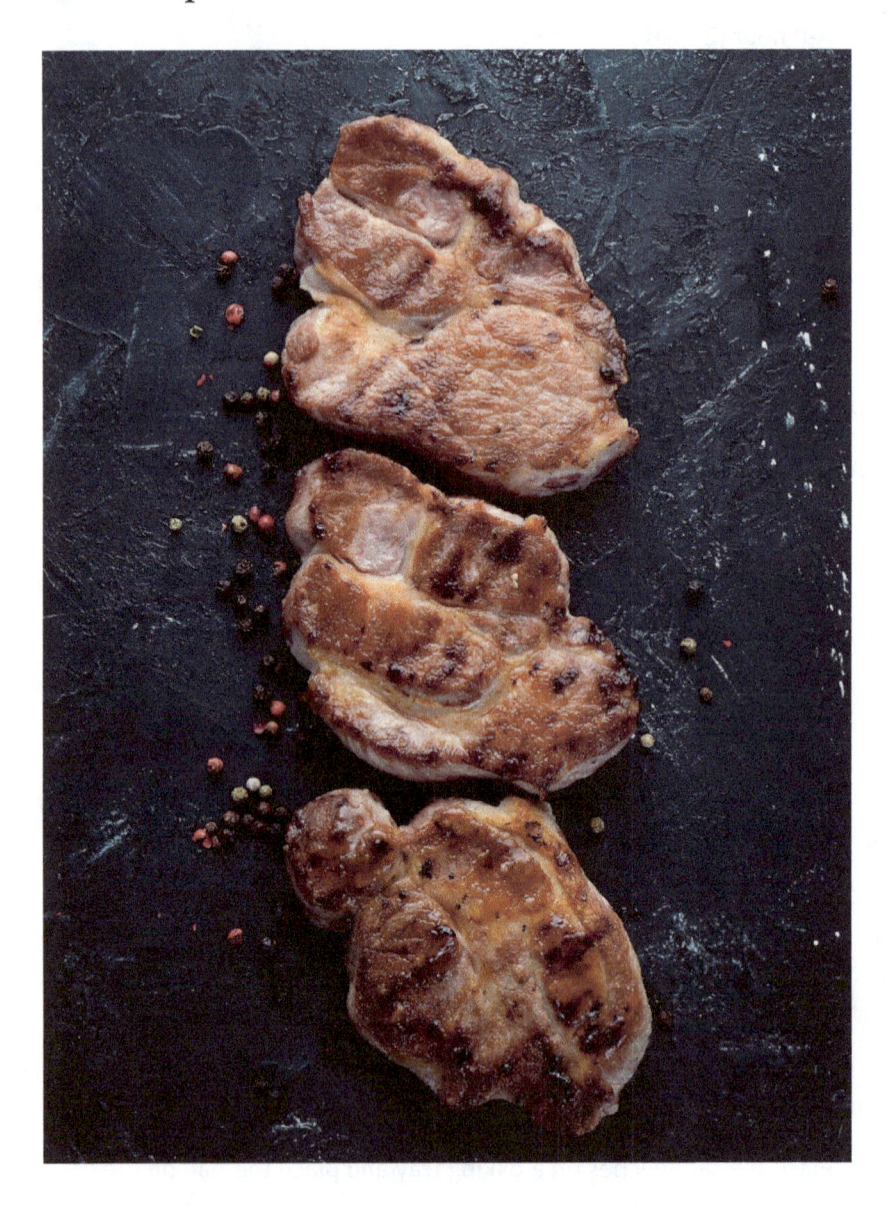

Servings Provided: 4

Time Required: 20 minutes

What is Needed:

- Olive oil (3 tbsp.)
- Boneless pork chops (4 - 1-inch or 1.5 lb.)
- Black pepper & kosher salt (.5 tsp. each/as desired)
- Finely chopped shallots (2)
- Dry white wine (.75 cup)
- Heavy cream (2 tbsp.)
- Dijon mustard (1 tbsp.)
- Freshly chopped tarragon (1 tbsp.)
- Torn frisée pieces (1 small head/4 cups)
- Lemon wedges (1)

Preparation Method:

1. Heat oven to 400° Fahrenheit.
2. Warm one tablespoon of the oil in a large skillet using the medium-high temperature setting.
3. Sprinkle the pork using pepper and salt. Let them cook and brown for two to three minutes per side.
4. Transfer the pork to a baking tray and roast until thoroughly cooked (5-7 min.).
5. Meanwhile, add the shallots and one tablespoon of the oil to the skillet and cook, often stirring, until softened (3-4 min.)
6. Add the wine to the skillet and simmer until reduced by half. Add the cream and simmer until the sauce just thickens. Stir in the mustard.
7. Top the pork with the sauce and tarragon. Drizzle the frisée with the remaining tablespoon of oil and serve with the lemon wedges.

Provencal Chicken Casserole

Servings Provided: 4

Time Required: 53 minutes

What is Needed:

- Olive oil (5 tbsp.)
- Chicken - broilers/fryers/breast - meat only (4 @ 6 oz.)
- Lemon juice (1 lemon)
- Table salt (1 pinch)
- Cherry tomatoes (1.5 cups)
- Onions - Spring/scallions - include tops & bulb (1 bunch)
- Swanson Clear Chicken Broth CAM (.5 cup)
- Brown mustard - prepared (2 tbsp.)
- Fresh rosemary (1.5 sprigs)
- Fresh thyme (half bunch)
- Cheese - gruyere (2 cups)

Preparation Method:

1. Pour three tablespoons of olive oil into a shallow platter and lay chicken breasts on top. Rub with lemon juice, salt, and pepper.
2. Warm two tablespoons of olive oil in a nonstick skillet using the med-high temperature function. Cook the chicken breasts until browned (4 min. per side).

3. Preheat the oven at 350° Fahrenheit. Grease a baking dish. Place tomatoes and green onions in the baking dish and pour the chicken broth on top.
4. Whisk the mustard, rosemary, and thyme in a small bowl and brush onto chicken breasts. Arrange the chicken breasts on top of the vegetables in the baking dish. Cover with the Gruyere cheese.
5. Bake the casserole on the middle rack until the chicken juices run clear and are no longer pink in the center (30 min.). (You can test it using an instant-read thermometer inserted into the center for a reading of at least 165° Fahrenheit.)

White Wine Coq Au Vin

Servings Provided: 6

Time Required: 55 minutes

What is Needed:

- Chicken - thighs, breasts & drumsticks (8 pieces/3 lb.)
- Black pepper & kosher salt
- Unsalted butter (2 tbsp.)
- Sliced bacon (4 diced)
- Large sweet onion (1)
- Garlic (3 minced cloves)
- Cremini mushrooms (1 pint - sliced)

- Dry white wine (2 cups)
- Whole-grain mustard (1 tbsp.)
- Heavy cream (.5 cup)
- Freshly chopped parsley (.25 cup)

Preparation Method:

1. Season the chicken with pepper and salt. Melt the butter in a large skillet using the medium temperature setting.
2. Arrange the chicken in the skillet and cook until it's well browned (4 min. per side).
3. Transfer the chicken from the skillet and set it aside. Add the bacon to the skillet and cook until the fat begins to render (3 min.).
4. Dice and mix in the onion and sauté until it is translucent (5 min.). Add the garlic and mushrooms, and sauté until the mushrooms are tender (5-6 min.).
5. Add the browned chicken back to the skillet. Pour the wine into the skillet, stir in the mustard, and bring the mixture to a simmer using the med-low temperature function. Cover the skillet and simmer until the chicken is almost fully cooked (15-20 min.).
6. Uncover the skillet and add the cream. Simmer until the sauce thickens and the chicken is fully cooked (8-10 min.).
7. Garnish with parsley and serve immediately.

PART IV

For all the meat lovers out there, the next diet that we are going to discuss is known as the carnivore diet.

Chapter 1: What Is Carnivore Diet?

The Carnivore Diet is the all-new trendy diet that expects its followers to go on a meat-only way of lifestyle. This diet completely goes against nutritional stereotyping. If someone asked you to replace that bowl of meat with vegetable oils and carbs, you probably have been misled!

This diet has won favor for several reasons and is, of course, not a fluke. If you find it attractive to sink in a carnivore way of eating, you have come to the right place.

The carnivore diet is the one that entirely revolves around a meat-based pattern of eating. It is one extreme diet that restricts you from eating plant-based foods and strictly opposes carbohydrate consumption. It might sound crazy, but there are people including Shawn Baker (the creator of this diet) who have normalized this fact that carbohydrate is a non-essential macronutrient, and there is no harm in cutting them down from the menu.

It is a zero-carb diet that altogether emphasizes consuming meat. Scientists consider this diet the best nutrition source for human beings, cutting out the chatter from plant toxins.

Science Behind Carnivore Diet: Reasons Why This Diet Will Work

There are more anecdotes and testimonials than research backed up with science. This no-carb diet has also been a second option to those who have either failed to carry on with Paleo and Keto diet or have faced other severe consequences after following them. This is a bold claim and has a lot to unpack. Let's dive deep into the depth of its science.

Researchers have carried out several studies throughout the Earth that has proved its benefits on humankind.

- **Removes the Inflammatory Vegetables** - If you have been suffering from an autoimmune disorder or a damaged gut, this might be of concern.

  Almost every vegetable has some kind of toxin in it. Brussels Sprouts, broccoli, cauliflower have sulforaphane that causes hypothyroidism and damage to health. Nightshades damage carb and fat metabolism. Polyphenols cause DNA damage. Lectins cause leaky guts. Reservatrol can inhibit androgen precursors. Spinach has oxalates that may result in kidney stones, and the list goes on. Choosing a carnivore diet can be a game-changing plan for such people and others who are still being manipulated by conventional nutritional advice.

- **It Increases Cholesterol** – You all must have heard about bad and good cholesterol. Cholesterol plays a negative role when it is oxidized or damaged and gets trapped in the artery walls. LDL cholesterol, even though it is given the tag of the 'bad' cholesterol, protects your body from diseases and does not cause them. They bind to the pathogens allowing the immune system to expel them.

During inflammation, the body uses LDL as a protective mechanism. So, people with heart diseases have high LDL levels because it binds to the pathogens, getting rid of the damage ensuring that it does not spread. It is, in fact, the inflammation that causes heart diseases.

- **It Increases the Nutrient Density** - Animal-based foods have the most bioavailable form of nutrients that play a crucial role from growth to brain function. While you have been a fiber-freak, you might just have missed out on the essential nutrients. Vegetarians have a deficiency in Vitamin B12 and Iron. Americans have Vitamin D deficiency, and women have Calcium deficiency, while Zinc is a deficient nutrient worldwide.

The brain requires micronutrients, and it is animals that mostly provide this. Zinc and iron are vital nutrients that help brain growth, dopamine transport, and serotonin synthesis.

- **It Reverses Insulin Resistance** - The best thing you could do to your health is reverse the insulin resistance. It is a problem where your body's cells become unresponsive to insulin action and therefore refuse to stuff the cells with more energy, leading to a rise in insulin level. It occurs due to excess carbohydrates and fat that shut off the process of burning fat, causing the fat to be stored without being used directly. The carnivore diet can be a solution to this!

- **Weight loss** - Since protein-based foods are satiating, they allow you to stay distracted from eating by making you feel fuller. By ingesting protein, the primary energy source is shifted from carbohydrate to fat. It is similar to ketosis (adapted to fat consumption), where you can use your body fat instead of carbohydrate.

How to Start the Diet?

Although it is as simple as a diet can be, the initial weeks can be hard. Here are the things that you can incorporate to get through the changeover conveniently:

- Before starting with the diet, you can get your blood test done since the metabolic needs vary with every individual.

- You might feel like giving up at some point, start getting headaches, and experience fatigue. It is normal as your body will be getting used to using energy from fat rather than carbohydrates.

- Your eating desire might fluctuate. You will get adjusted to this form of eating after one week.

Chapter 2: Recipes for Tasty Appetizers

If you are a meat lover and want to start the carnivore diet, here are some recipes for you to follow.

Oven-Baked Chicken Wings

Total Prep & Cooking Time: 1 hour 5 minutes

Yields: 8 servings

Nutrition Facts: Calories: 348 | Carbs: 1g | Protein: 25g | Fat: 27g | Fiber: 1g

Ingredients:

- Half cup of grated Parmesan
- Four pounds of chicken wings
- One tsp. of salt
- One tbsp. of parsley
- A quarter cup of grass-fed butter
- Half tsp. of black pepper (ground)

Method:

1. First of all, the oven needs to be preheated to 180 degrees Celsius or 350 degrees Fahrenheit.

2. Take a parchment paper for lining the baking sheet.

3. Now, you need to take a shallow bowl or dish for melting the butter.

4. In another clean bowl, mix parsley, pepper, Parmesan cheese, and salt.

5. Once the herb and cheese mixture is ready, dip the chicken wings in the bowl of melted butter one by one. After dipping, roll the wings in the mixture.

6. Arrange all the wings properly on top of the baking sheet.

7. Bake for an hour.

8. Take out the baked chicken wings from the oven and serve them warm.

Steak Nuggets

Total Prep & Cooking Time: 55-60 minutes

Yields: 4 servings

Nutrition Facts: Calories: 350 | Carbs: 1g | Protein: 40g | Fat: 20g | Fiber: 2g

Ingredients:

- One pound of beefsteak or venison steak (cut it into chunks)
- Palm or lard oil (needed for frying)
- One large-sized egg

For Keto Breading,

- Half cup each of
  - Pork panko
  - Parmesan cheese (grated)
- Half tsp. of seasoned salt (homemade)

For Chipotle Ranch Dip,

- A quarter cup each of
  - Organic cultured cream (sour)
  - Mayonnaise
- More than one tsp. of chipotle paste (for taste)
- A quarter medium-sized lime (juiced)

Method:

1. For preparing the Chipotle Ranch Dip, you need to combine all the ingredients and mix properly. Use either more or less chipotle paste in accordance to your taste preference. Refrigerate the dip before serving for a minimum of thirty minutes. You may store the dip for nearly a week.

2. Take a large-sized bowl and combine parmesan cheese, seasoned salt, and pork panko. Set aside after mixing evenly.

3. Now, beat one egg. Place the breading mix in one bowl and beaten egg in another.

4. Dip the steak chunks first in egg and then in the breading mix. Then, place them on a plate or sheet pan lined with wax paper.

5. Before frying, freeze the raw breaded steak bites for half an hour. By doing so, the breading won't lift at the time of frying.

6. Heat the lard to 325 degrees Fahrenheit. Fry the chilled or frozen steak nuggets for nearly two to three minutes until you get the brown color.

7. Keep the fried nuggets on a plate lined with a paper towel. Sprinkle a pinch of salt. Serve hot along with Chipotle Ranch.

Grilled Shrimp

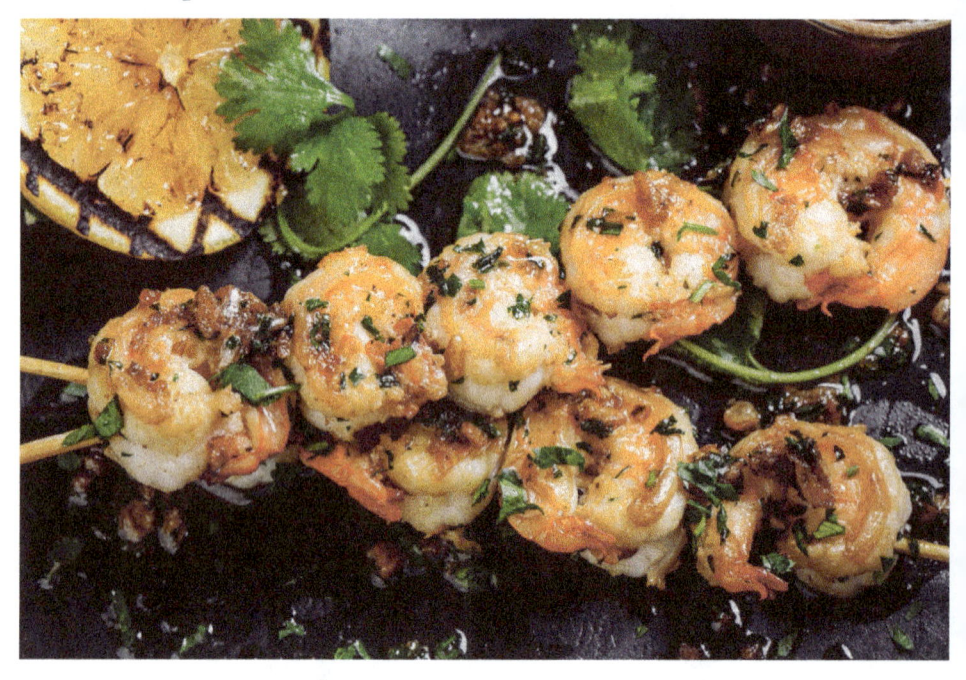

Total Prep & Cooking Time: 10 minutes

Yields: 4 servings

Nutrition Facts: Calories: 102 | Carbs: 1g | Protein: 28g | Fat: 3g | Fiber: 0g

Ingredients:

For grilling,

- One lb. of shrimp
- One tbsp. of lemon juice (freshly squeezed)

- Two tbsps. of olive oil (extra-virgin)
- For frying – vegetable oil or canola oil

For the shrimp seasoning,

- Half a tsp. of cayenne pepper
- One tsp. each of
    - Italian seasoning
    - Kosher salt
    - Garlic powder

Method:

1. You have to preheat your grill for this recipe on high.

2. Take a mixing bowl of large size, add all the ingredients of the seasoning in it and mix them well. Drizzle the lemon juice and olive oil into the mixture and keep stirring until you get a paste.

3. Add the shrimp into the bowl of seasonings and keep tossing so that all the pieces are evenly coated. Take the shrimp pieces and thread them onto wooden skewers.

4. Coat your grill with canola oil. You have to grill the shrimp for about three minutes for each side until they become opaque and pink.

5. Serve and enjoy!

Notes: *You can store the grilled shrimp in the refrigerator for up to three days if you want to, but for the best flavor, you should consume it on the same day.*

Roasted Bone Marrow

Total Prep & Cooking Time: 20 minutes

Yields: 2 servings

Nutrition Facts: Calories: 440 | Carbs: 0g | Protein: 4g | Fat: 48g | Fiber: 0g

Ingredients:

- To season – freshly ground black pepper and sea salt flakes
- Four bone marrow halves

Method:

1. Set the temperature of your oven to 350 degrees F and preheat.
2. Take a baking tray with deep sides and then place the bone marrow pieces in it.
3. Bake the bone marrow for half an hour until they become crispy and golden brown in color. The fat that is present in excess should have rendered off by now.
4. Season with black pepper and sea salt flakes.
5. You can spread the marrow separately on top of steaks, or you can serve the bone marrow as an appetizer.

Bacon-Wrapped Chicken Bites

Total Prep & Cooking Time: 30 minutes

Yields: 4 servings

Nutrition Facts: Calories: 230 | Carbs: 5g | Protein: 22g | Fat: 13g | Fiber: 1g

Ingredients:

- Three tbsps. of garlic powder
- Eight slices of thin bacon (slice them into one-third pieces)
- One chicken breast (large-sized, cut into bite-sized pieces)

Method:

1. Set the temperature of the oven to 400 degrees F and use aluminum foil to line the baking tray—Preheat the oven.

2. In a bowl, add the garlic powder. Take each chicken piece and dip it into the garlic powder.

3. Now, take each short piece of bacon and wrap it around the piece of chicken. Keep these prepared chicken pieces on the baking tray. Make sure they are not touching each other.

4. Bake the preparation for half an hour, and by the end of it, the bacon should turn crispy. After about fifteen minutes through pieces, turn the pieces over.

Salami Egg Muffins

Total Prep & Cooking Time: 25 minutes

Yields: 12 servings

Nutrition Facts: Calories: 142 | Carbs: 1g | Protein: 12g | Fat: 10g | Fiber: 0g

Ingredients:

- Four eggs (large-sized)
- Twenty slices of salami (uncured)
- Half a tsp. of kosher salt
- A quarter tsp. of black pepper
- Olive oil

Method:

1. Set the temperature of the oven to 350 degrees F and preheat. Take ramekins of four ounces each and spray them with olive oil. Then, place these ramekins on the baking sheet.

2. On the bottom of each ramekin, place one slice of salami and then on the sides, arrange four slices so that they are overlapping each other.

3. In this way, you will get a basket of salami, and in the middle of the basket, break one egg. Form four such baskets. Season the baskets with pepper and salt.

4. Bake the prepared salami baskets for twenty minutes, and by that time, they should be set.

5. Around the edges of the muffins, run a knife, and the muffins will get released. Serve and enjoy!

3-Ingredients Scotch Eggs

Total Prep & Cooking Time: 40 minutes

Yields: 12 servings

Nutrition Facts: Calories: 270 | Carbs: 1g | Protein: 19g | Fat: 20g | Fiber: 5g

Ingredients:

- Twelve large-sized boiled eggs
- Two pounds of chicken sausage or ground beef
- Two tsps. of salt

Method:

1. Preheating the oven to a temperature of 175 degrees Celsius or 350 degrees Fahrenheit is the first step for preparing such a delicious appetizer.
2. Line two baking sheets (small rimmed) with a parchment paper.
3. Take a large-sized bowl and combine chicken or beef and salt. Mix both the ingredients together by using your hands and then form twelve meatballs with it. Press the meatballs flat after placing them on top of the lined sheets.

4. Now, place each boiled egg inside each circle of flattened meat. After placing the eggs, start wrapping the meat nicely around the eggs. You are not supposed to leave any holes or gaps.

5. You need to bake for nearly fifteen minutes. Flip over as soon as the top looks cooked and again bake for ten minutes. If you want a crispy shell, then finish it under a broiler for approximately five minutes.

Notes: *If you are willing to enhance the taste, then you may feel free to add any of your favorite herbs, such as garlic or rosemary powder. Add one tsp. of your preferred herb into the meat just before wrapping the eggs. Hard-boiled eggs are better in this case as it is difficult to peel the soft boiled eggs.*

Chapter 3: Quick and Easy Everyday Recipes

Carnivore Waffles

Total Prep & Cooking Time: 6 minutes

Yields: 1 serving

Nutrition Facts: Calories: 274 | Carbs: 1g | Protein: 23.6g | Fat: 20.2g | Fiber: 0.8g

Ingredients:

- One-third cup of mozzarella cheese
- One egg
- Half cup of pork rinds (ground)
- A pinch of salt

Method:

1. For preparing the carnivore waffles, all you need is a waffle maker. First of all, preheat your waffle maker (medium-high heat).

2. Take a medium-sized bowl and whisk the pork rinds, cheese, and salt together.

3. Once you are done with the whisking part, pour the already prepared waffle mixture in the middle of the waffle maker's iron.

4. Close it and allow it to cook for three to five minutes. Or, you may cook until the waffle gets an attractive golden brown color.

5. Now, remove the cooked waffle and serve hot.

Notes: *The carnivore waffle will turn out to be more delicious if you place a cube of butter or runny egg on top of it. Greasing the waffle maker is not required before you start cooking waffles.*

Chicken Bacon Pancakes

Total Prep & Cooking Time: 20 minutes

Yields: 4 servings

Nutrition Facts: Calories: 444 | Carbs: 0g | Protein: 33g | Fat: 34g | Fiber: 0g

Ingredients:

- Four bacon slices
- Two chicken breasts
- Two tbsps. of coconut oil
- Four eggs (medium-sized, whisked)

Method:

1. First, you need to add all the ingredients to the bowl of the food processor except for the oil and then process everything together to form a smooth mixture.
2. After that, take your frying pan, and coconut oil to it.
3. From the batter that you just made, form four pancakes.
4. Fry these pancakes until they are set and properly cooked. Do the same with the rest of the batter.

Garlic Cilantro Salmon

Total Prep & Cooking Time: 25 minutes

Yields: 4 servings

Nutrition Facts: Calories: 294 | Carbs: 1g | Protein: 38.9g | Fat: 14.2g | Fiber: 0g

Ingredients:

- One lemon
- One fillet of salmon (large)
- A quarter cup of cilantro leaves (freshly chopped)
- Four garlic cloves (minced)
- One tablespoon of butter (optional)
- To taste – freshly ground black pepper and kosher salt

Method:

1. Set the temperature of the oven to 400 degrees F and preheat. Take a baking sheet and line it with foil. Place the fillets of salmon on it. You don't have to grease the foil.

2. Sprinkle the juice of one lemon over the fillet of salmon. Spread cilantro and garlic on top of the fillets evenly and season with pepper and salt. If you want to use butter, then you have to place thin slices on top of the salmon fillet at this stage.

3. Now, place the salmon along with the foil in the oven and bake for about seven minutes.

4. Set broil settings and cook the salmon for an additional seven minutes. The top part should become crispy.

5. Use a flat spatula to remove the salmon from the oven. Separate the skin from the fish and serve!

Mustard-Seared Bacon Burgers

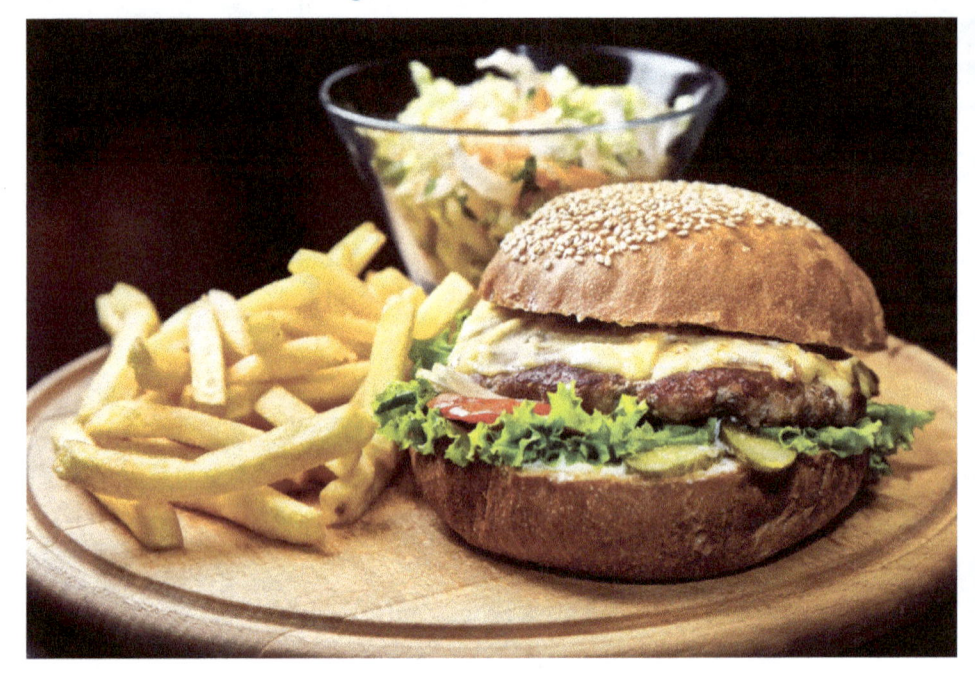

Total Prep & Cooking Time: 30 minutes

Yields: 6 servings

Nutrition Facts: Calories: 525 | Carbs: 3g | Protein: 22g | Fat: 45g | Fiber: 4g

Ingredients:

- 1.5 pounds of ground beef
- Four ounces of diced bacon
- Six tbsps. of yellow mustard
- To taste – salt and pepper

For the toppings,

- One tomato (properly diced)
- Half a red onion (diced)
- One avocado (thinly sliced)

For the sauce,

- Two tsps. of yellow mustard
- One tsp. of tomato paste
- A quarter cup of mayo

Method:

1. Take a pan and cook the bacon in it until it becomes crispy. You have to keep the grease of the bacon separately so that it can be used later. Then, take the bacon bits and keep them in a bowl along with the ground beef. Use pepper and salt to season them.

2. You will be able to form six patties from the mixture.

3. Now, you have to fry these burger patties on high flame so that they can get a great color. If you want, you can also choose to grill them.

4. Each patty will then have to be coated with one tbsp. of mustard and then, place the patty on the pan with the mustard-side facing down. Sear the patties one by one.

5. Take another bowl in which you can mix all the ingredients of the sauce together.

6. Each burger patty will have to be coated with sauce, and then, you can top them with slices of avocado, tomato, and onions.

Crockpot Shredded Chicken

Total Prep & Cooking Time: 6 hours

Yields: 8 servings

Nutrition Facts: Calories: 201 | Carbs: 1g | Protein: 24g | Fat: 10g | Fiber: 0g

Ingredients:

- Four garlic cloves
- Four chicken breasts
- One cup of chicken broth
- Half an onion (sliced)
- One tbsp. of Italian seasoning
- To taste – Salt and pepper

Method:

1. Take all the ingredients and add them to the crockpot.
2. Cook them for about six hours on low.
3. Use forks to shred the meat.
4. You can enjoy the shredded chicken with a variety of dishes like sautés, lettuce wraps, salads, or even soups.

Chapter 4: Weekend Dinner Recipes

Organ Meat Pie
Total Prep & Cooking Time: 20 minutes

Yields: 4 servings

Nutrition Facts: Calories: 412 | Carbs: 2g | Protein: 35g | Fat: 28g | Fiber: 4.2g

Ingredients:

- Half pound each of
    - Beef liver (ground)
    - Beef heart (ground)
    - Ground beef
- Three eggs
- Butter, ghee or Homemade Tallow or any melted cooking fat
- Salt (as required)

Method:

1. The oven needs to be preheated to 175 degrees Celsius or 350 degrees Fahrenheit.

2. Take a mixing bowl: mix ground beef, beef heart, and beef liver along with eggs and cooking fat of your choice. Lastly, add salt into the mixture.

3. Now, take a pie plate of nine inches and grease it lightly. Pour the mixture into the pie plate evenly.

4. Bake it for nearly fifteen to twenty minutes. Or, you may bake until the egg is totally set.

5. After baking, remove the pie from direct heat and let it cool for about five minutes. Serve it in a warm condition. In the case of leftovers, enjoy it cold.

Notes: *For those of you who are willing to add flavor to this recipe, you may add half tbsp. of any seasoning mix with the meat.*

Smokey Bacon Meatballs

Total Prep & Cooking Time: 30 minutes

Yields: 8 servings

Nutrition Facts: Calories: 280 | Carbs: 1g | Protein: 13g | Fat: 25g | Fiber: 0g

Ingredients:

- Two garlic cloves (skins peeled)
- Eight bacon slices (crumbled and cooked)
- One pound ground chicken or two chicken breasts
- One egg (properly whisked)
- Two drops of liquid smoke
- One tbsp. of onion powder
- Four tbsps. of olive oil

Method:

1. First, take all the ingredients (except for the oil) and add them to the bowl of the food processor and mix everything.

2. You will be able to form about twenty to twenty-four meatballs from the mixture. These balls will be small in size.

3. Now, take a large-sized frying pan, and then heat the oil. Add the meatballs and fry them until they are browned. It will take about five minutes for each side. If you want them to be perfect, then avoid overcrowding and cook in batches.

Steak au Poivre

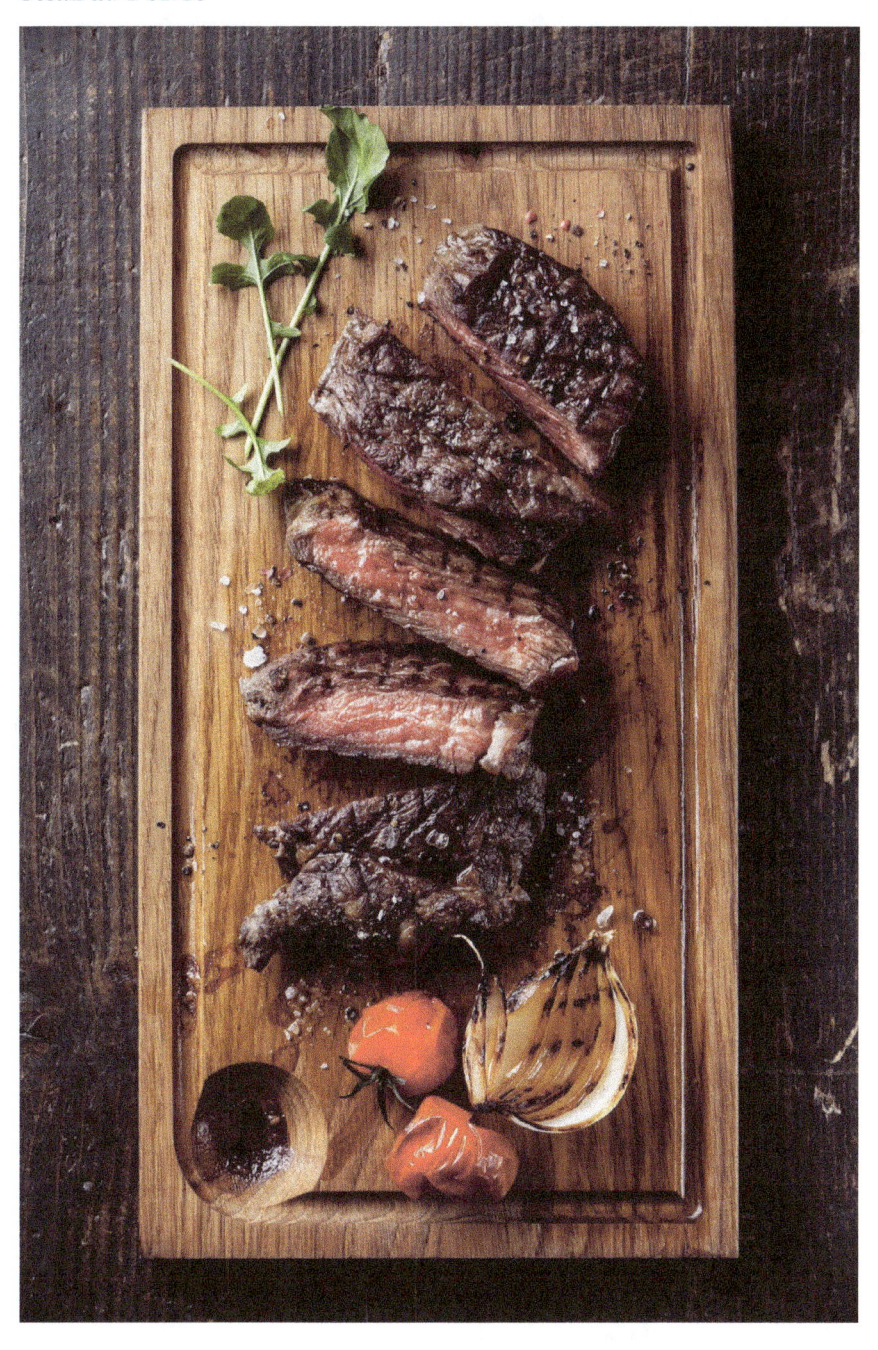

Total Prep & Cooking Time: 15 minutes

Yields: 1 serving

Nutrition Facts: Calories: 696 | Carbs: 2g | Protein: 42g | Fat: 58g | Fiber: 0g

Ingredients:

- One fillet of mignon (approximately six ounces)
- One thyme sprig
- One tbsp. of salt
- Two tbsps. each of
  - Ghee
  - Peppercorns
- Two garlic cloves (minced)

Method:

1. After you take the steaks out of the refrigerator, season them nicely with salt and then allow them to sit for about half an hour.

2. Use a mortar and pestle to crush the peppercorns completely on a pan or a flat board.

3. Take the steak, and on both sides of it, press the crushed peppercorns.

4. Place a skillet on the oven and heat it. Add the ghee. After that, sauté the thyme and garlic.

5. When you notice that the ghee has become hot, place the pieces of steak in the pan. Cook each side for about four minutes. The end result will be medium-rare steak.

Skillet Rib Eye Steaks

Total Prep & Cooking Time: 55 minutes

Yields: 2 servings

Nutrition Facts: Calories: 347 | Carbs: 1g | Protein: 22g | Fat: 14.2g | Fiber: 0g

Ingredients:

- Two tsps. of freshly chopped rosemary leaves
- One tsp. of seasoning of your choice
- One tbsp. each of
  - Olive oil
  - Unsalted butter
- One rib-eye steak (bone-in)

Method:

1. Take the sheet pan and on it, place the rib-eye steak. Use the seasoning to coat both sides properly. Spread the rosemary leaves on top.

2. Now, keep this steak in the refrigerator for three days after covering. Before cooking, take the steak out and keep it outside at room temperature for half an hour.

3. Place a skillet on the oven and heat it. Add olive oil and butter and wait until all of the butter has melted. Coat the skillet properly with butter by tilting the pan.

4. Now, add the steak to the skillet and cook for about five minutes until you notice that the bottom side has become caramelized and browned. After that, flip it over and baste the other side with oil and butter and cook it for five more minutes.

5. Take the steak off from the pan and slice it into thin pieces after it has cooled down for about five minutes.

Pan-Fried Pork Tenderloin

Total Prep & Cooking Time: 20 minutes

Yields: 2 servings

Nutrition Facts: Calories: 330 | Carbs: 0g | Protein: 47g | Fat: 15g | Fiber: 0g

Ingredients:

- One tbsp. of coconut oil
- To taste – pepper and salt
- One pound of pork tenderloin

Method:

1. Start by cutting the pork tenderloin in two halves.
2. Place your frying pan on the oven on medium flame. Add the oil in the pan and heat it.
3. Once the oil has melted completely, place the two pieces of the pork tenderloin in the oil.
4. Allow the pieces to cook thoroughly. Use tongs to flip the pieces so that all the sides of the pork are evenly cooked.
5. Take a reading on the thermometer, and it should show that the temperature is just below 63 degrees C or 145 degrees F.
6. Allow the pork to cool down after you take it out and then use a sharp knife to cut it into small pieces.

Carnivore Chicken Enchiladas

Total Prep & Cooking Time: 30 minutes

Yields: 10 servings

Nutrition Facts: Calories: 271 | Carbs: 5g | Protein: 25g | Fat: 7g | Fiber: 1.5g

Ingredients:

- Two chicken breasts (skinless, boneless)
- Three tbsps. of bottles lime juice + juice of one fresh lime
- One tsp. of dried garlic
- 16 oz. of sliced chicken
- Chimichurri sauce
- One jar of enchilada sauce
- One bell pepper (thinly sliced)
- Eight oz. each of
    - Cooked spinach
    - Shredded cheese

Method:

For making the shredded chicken,

1. First, take a crockpot and add the shredded pieces of chicken in it. Add the lime juice too.

2. Sprinkle the Chimichurri sauce on top of the chicken and then sprinkle the garlic on top.

3. Now, cook the chicken for about 4-5 hours if you want to cook it on high. Alternatively, if you're going to cook it on low, then set it for 8 hours.

4. Once it is done, use a fork to shred the chicken.

Assembling the enchiladas,

1. Set the temperature of your oven to 400 degrees F and preheat.

2. Take all the other ingredients like pepper and spinach and prep them.

3. The enchilada wrapped will be made by the four slices of chicken.

4. In the middle of the wrapper, add the shredded chicken.

5. Then, on either side, add the cooked spinach, pepper, and some of the cheese.

6. Roll the wrappers carefully and make sure they are firm.

7. Once you have rolled them completely, place them in a pan with the seam sides facing downwards. Then, add the enchilada sauce all over them.

8. Take the remaining portion of the cheese and sprinkle on top of the enchiladas. Bake the preparation for about fifteen minutes in the oven.

9. Serve and enjoy!

PART V

Before we get started on your new recipes, let's learn how to make a delicious rub for your favorite meat.

Grilling Rub

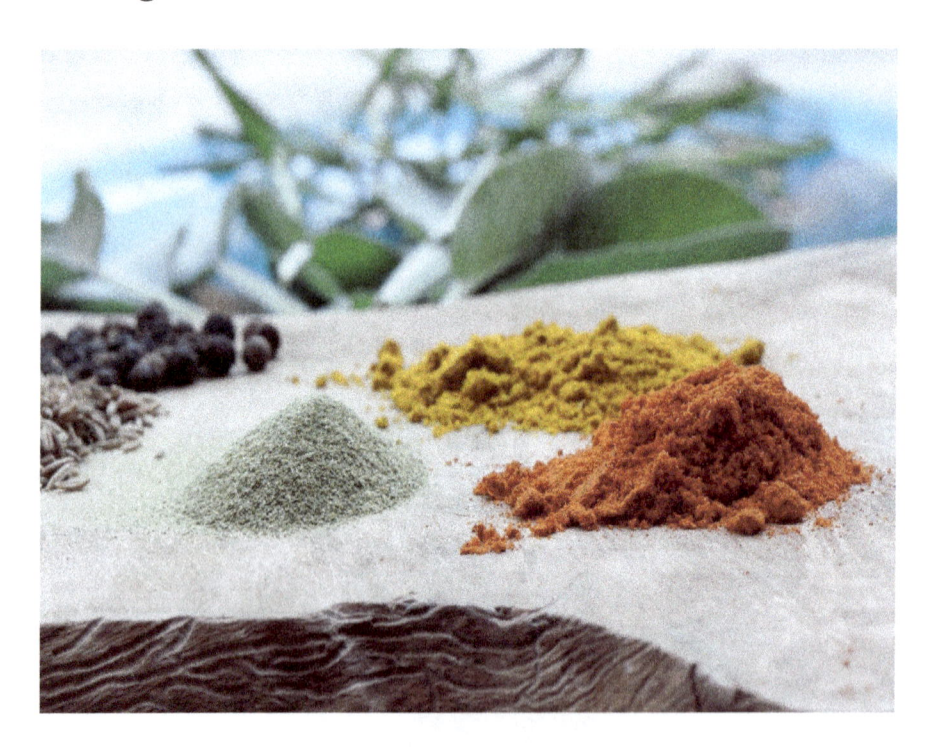

What is Needed:

- Finely ground dark-roast coffee (3 tbsp.)
- Chili powder (3 tbsp.)
- Chipotle powder (1 tsp.)
- Dark brown sugar (3 tbsp.)
- Kosher salt (2 tbsp.)

- Smoked paprika (2 tbsp.)
- Dried thyme (1 tbsp.)
- Granulated garlic (1 tbsp.)
- Ground cumin (2 tsp.)

Preparation Method:

1. Be sure to pack the sugar when it's measured - tightly. Combine each of the fixings and rub them into the chosen meat.
2. Leave the rub on the meat for 12-24 hours before grilling.

Chapter 1: Seafood

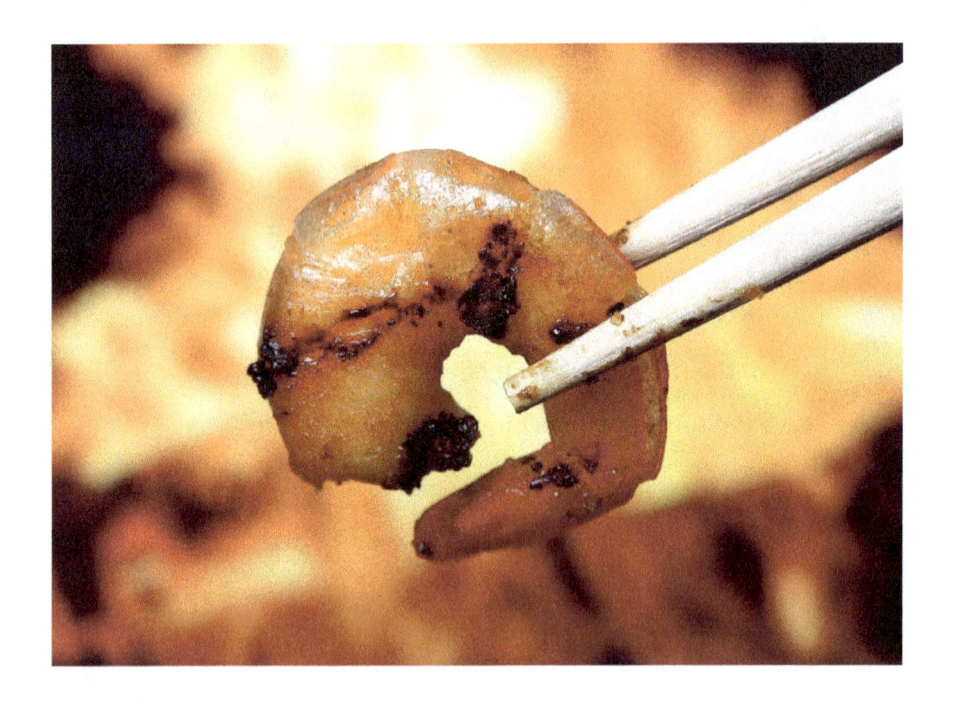

Lemony Shrimp & Tomatoes

Servings Provided: 4 kabobs with ½ cup sauce each

Time Required: 25 minutes

What is Needed:

- Olive oil (2 tbsp.)
- Lemon juice (.33 cup)
- Grated lemon zest (.5 tsp.)
- Uncooked jumbo shrimp (1 lb.)
- Fresh arugula (2/3 cup)

- Sliced green onions (2)
- Plain yogurt (.25 cup)
- 2% milk (2 tsp.)
- Cider vinegar (1 tsp.)
- Sugar (.5 tsp.)
- Garlic (2 cloves)
- Dijon mustard (1 tsp.)
- Salt (.5 tsp. divided)
- Cherry tomatoes (12)
- Pepper (.25 tsp.)
- Also Needed: Skewers (4)

Preparation Method:

1. If you plan to use wooden skewers, be sure to soak them in water before you thread them.
2. Prepare a large mixing container and add the lemon juice, oil, minced garlic, and lemon zest, whisking until blended.
3. Fold in the shrimp and wait for about ten minutes.
4. Rinse and toss the arugula, green onions, yogurt, milk, vinegar, mustard, sugar, and ¼ of teaspoon salt in a food processor, pulsing until smooth.
5. Peel and devein the shrimp.
6. Prepare the skewers by alternating using the shrimp and tomatoes. Sprinkle it with pepper and rest of the salt.
7. Grill, covered, using the med-high temperature setting for two to three minutes per side or until shrimp are no longer pink.
8. Serve the kabobs with sauce.

Sea Bass With Garlic Butter

Servings Provided: 4

Time Required: 25 minutes

What is Needed:

- Sea bass (2 lb.)
- Butter (3 tbsp.)
- Lemon juice (1 medium lemon)
- Italian parsley (2 tbsp.)
- Olive oil (1.5 tbsp.)
- Cloves of garlic (2)

    Spices - .25 tsp. each:

- Garlic powder
- Paprika
- Onion powder
- Sea salt

Preparation Method:

1. Mince the garlic and finely chop the parsley.
2. Make the sauce. Prepare a saucepan to melt the butter and combine it with the lemon juice, garlic, and parsley. Transfer the pan to a cool burner once the butter has melted.

3. Warm the grill using the med-high temperature setting.
4. Oil the grates right before placing the fish onto the grill.
5. Combine the garlic, onion powder, paprika, pepper, and salt in a small mixing bowl.
6. Sprinkle the seasoning mixture on each side of the fish.
7. Grill the sea bass for seven minutes. Turn the fish and coat it with the butter sauce. Grill it for about seven additional minutes.
8. Once the fish reaches an internal temperature of at least 145° Fahrenheit, remove it from the heat, and spritz it with olive oil.
9. Serve it with your favorite sides.

Chapter 2: Pork

Grilled Sausages With Summer Veggies

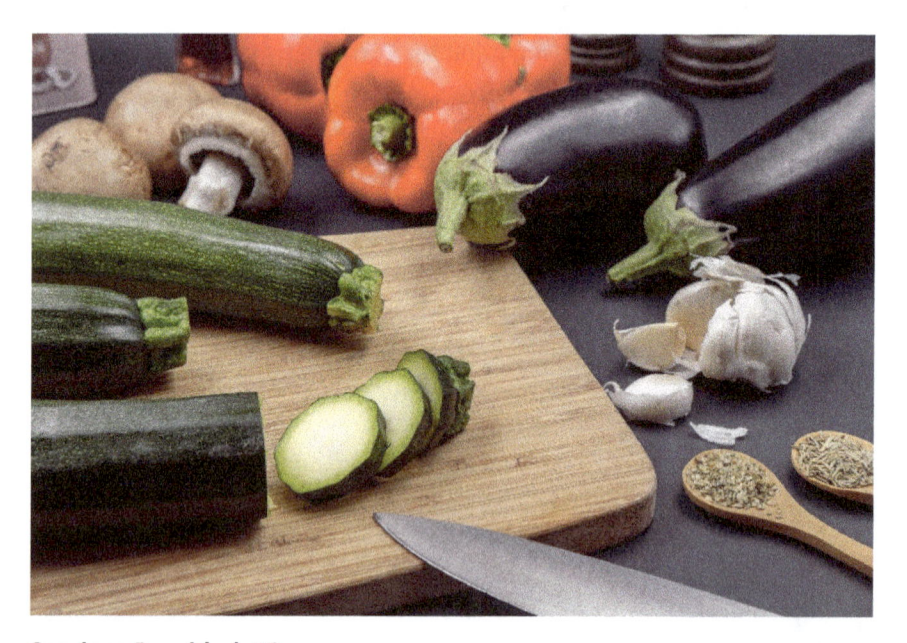

Servings Provided: 12

Time Required: 60 minutes

What is Needed:

- Peach preserves (.75 cup)
- Soy sauce (.5 cup)
- Freshly minced ginger root (.5 cup)
- Water (3 tbsp.)

- Garlic (3 minced cloves)
- Optional: Hot pepper sauce (1 dash)
- Sweet red peppers (4 medium)
- Zucchini (3 small)
- Eggplant (1 medium)
- Yellow summer squash (2 small)
- Italian pork/turkey sausage links (12 hot @ 4 oz. each)

Preparation Method:

1. Measure and add the first five ingredients (up to the line) in a blender, adding the pepper sauce as desired. Cover with the lid and mix until blended.
2. Slice the zucchini and yellow squash lengthwise into quarters. Slice the peppers lengthwise in half and remove the seeds. Cut eggplant lengthwise into 1/2-inch-thick slices. Place all vegetables in a big mixing container and drizzle them using ½ cup of the sauce and toss to coat.
3. Place the veggies onto a greased grill rack. Grill, covered using medium heat until tender and lightly charred, turning once (8-10 min.). Cool slightly and adjust the grill temperature to the med-low setting.
4. Cut vegetables into bite-sized pieces. Toss with an additional ¼ cup sauce and keep warm.
5. Grill the sausages, covered, on med-low heat setting for 15-20 minutes or until a thermometer reads 160° Fahrenheit for pork

sausages (165° Fahrenheit for turkey sausages) - turning occasionally. Remove sausages from grill and toss with the remaining sauce. Serve with vegetables.

Honey-Chipotle Ribs

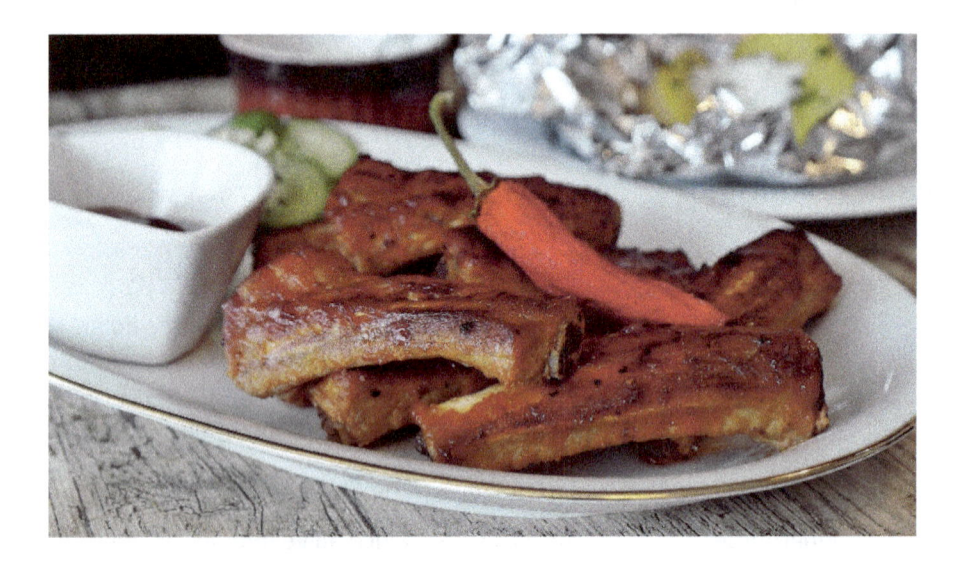

Servings Provided: 12

Time Required: 1 hour 35 minutes

What is Needed:

- Pork baby back ribs (6 lb.)
  The Sauce:

- Ground chipotle pepper (4 tsp.)
- Chipotle peppers - in adobo sauce (2 tbsp.)
- Guinness beer (2 bottles - 11.2 oz ea.)
- Ketchup (3 cups)
- BBQ sauce (2 cups)
- Honey (2/3 cup)
- Onion (1 small)
- Worcestershire sauce (.25 cup)
- Dijon mustard (2 tbsp.)
- Black pepper (.5 tsp.)
- Salt (1 tsp.)
- Garlic powder (1 tsp.)

Preparation Method:

1. Chop the onion and chipotle peppers.
2. Wrap the ribs in large pieces of heavy-duty foil, sealing the edges of foil.
3. Grill the ribs with the lid 'on' while using indirect medium heat until tender (1-1.5 hrs.).
4. Combine the sauce ingredients in a large saucepan.
5. Adjust the temperature setting to simmer, uncovered, for about 45 minutes - until thickened - stirring occasionally.
6. Remove ribs from foil and place over direct heat. Baste them with some of the sauce.

7. Grill the ribs with the lid on, using the medium temperature setting for about half an hour or until browned, turning once and occasionally basting with additional sauce.
8. Serve with the rest of the sauce.

Peachy Pork Ribs

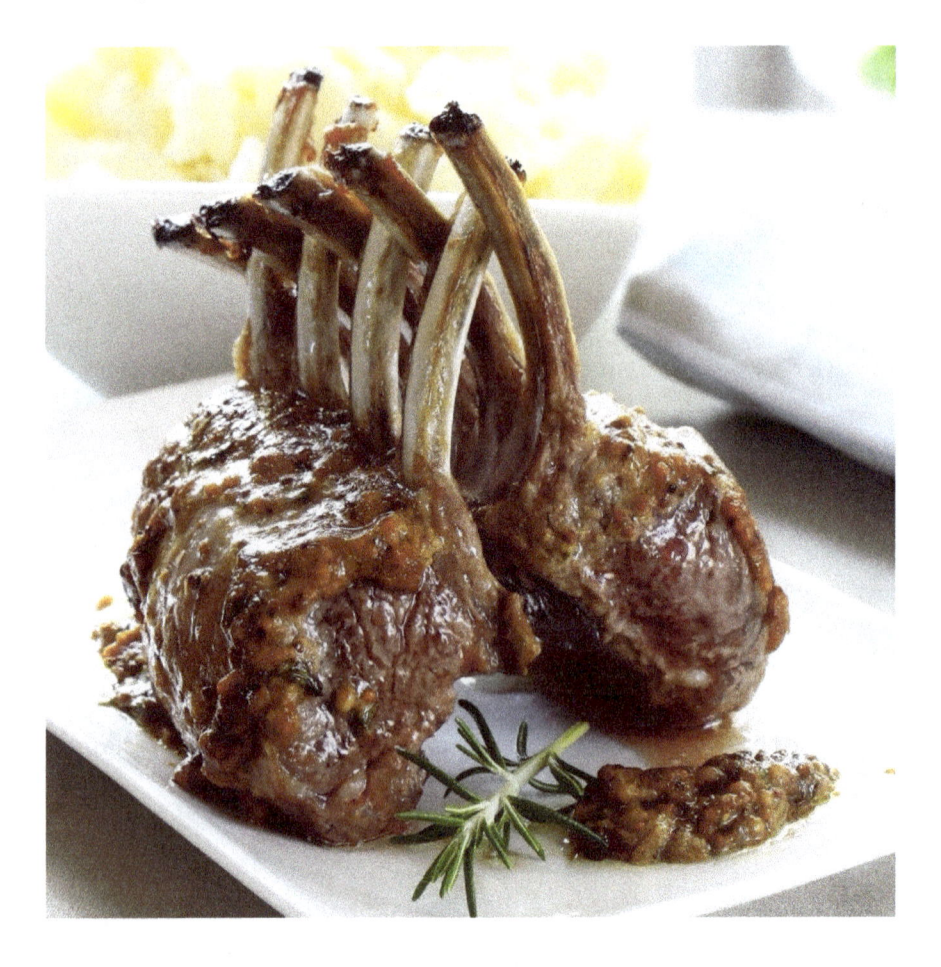

Servings Provided: 4

Time Required: 2.5 hours

What is Needed:

- Pork baby back ribs (4 lb./in serving-sized portions)
- Water (.5 cup)
- Ripe peaches (3 medium)
- Onion (2 tbsp.)
- Butter (2 tbsp.)
- Garlic (1 clove)
- Lemon juice (3 tbsp.)
- Orange juice concentrate (2 tbsp.)
- Soy sauce (2 tsp.)
- Ground mustard (.5 tsp.)
- Brown sugar (1 tbsp.)
- Salt (.25 tsp.)

Preparation Method:

1. Mince the garlic and onion.
2. Add the ribs into a shallow roasting pan of water.
3. Place a layer of foil over the pan, and bake at 325° Fahrenheit for two hours.
4. Peel and cube the peaches and toss them into a blender, cover, and process until blended.
5. Prepare a small saucepan to melt the butter. Sauté the onion until tender. Mix in the garlic and sauté for one more minute. Stir in the lemon juice, orange juice concentrate, soy sauce, brown sugar, mustard, pepper, salt, and pureed peaches. Warm until thoroughly heated.
6. Drain the ribs. Spoon some of the sauce over ribs.
7. Grill the ribs using the medium temperature setting on a lightly oiled rack, covered, for eight to ten minutes or until browned, turning occasionally and brushing with sauce.

Pork Loin Steaks

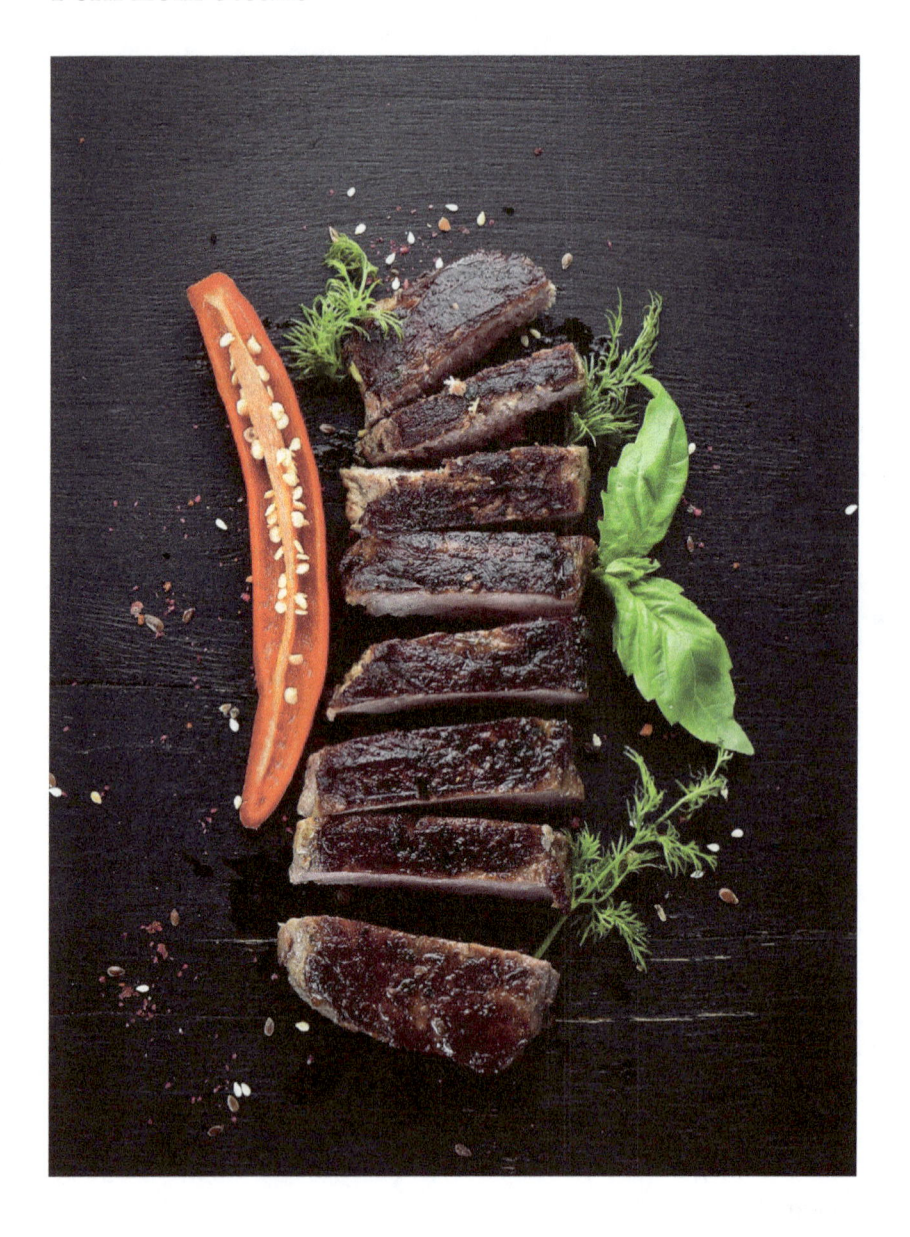

Servings Provided: 2

Time Required: 25 minutes

What is Needed:

- Pork loin steaks (4 boneless)
- Water (.25 cup)
- Dried oregano (1 tsp.)
- Brown sugar (2 tbsp.)

Preparation Method:

1. Use a non-metallic container to combine the marinade fixings.
2. Add the steaks to the bowl and cover to marinate overnight or for a minimum of two hours in the fridge.
3. Prepare the grill using the med-high temperature setting.
4. Grill the steaks for three to five minutes on each side and serve with your favorite side dishes.

Chapter 3: Poultry

Chicago-Style Turkey Dogs

Servings Provided: 4

Time Required: 20 minutes

What is Needed:

- Turkey hot dogs (4)
- Whole wheat tortillas (4 @ 8-inch - warmed)
- Sandwich pickle slices (4 thin)
- Chopped sweet onions (.5 cup)
- Optional Toppings:
- Prepared mustard
- Pickled hot peppers
- Cheddar cheese

Preparation Method:

1. Grill the hot dogs until they are as you like them - with the grill marks.
2. Serve in a tortilla with a portion of tomatoes, cucumber, pickles, and onions.
3. Add more toppings as desired.

Dr. Pepper Drumsticks

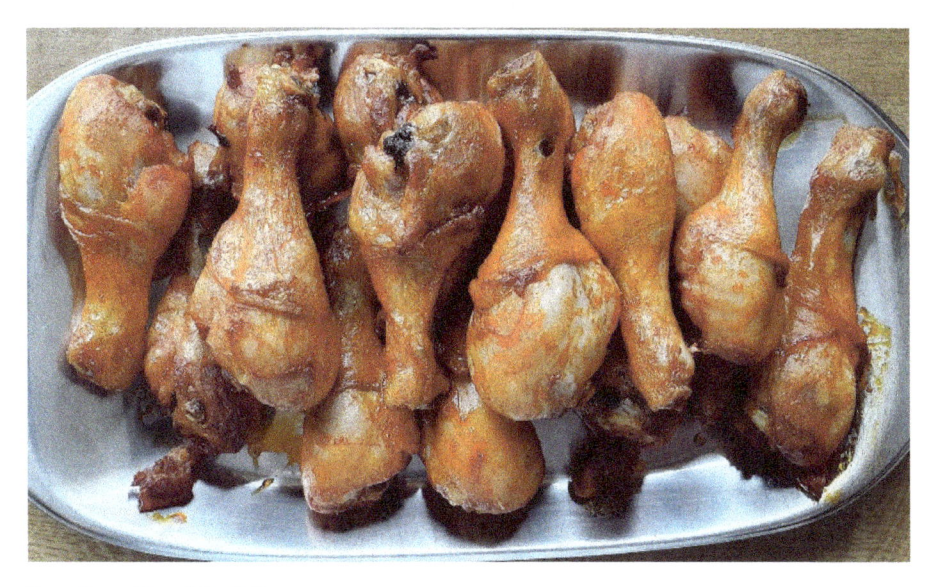

Servings Provided: 6

Time Required: 50 minutes

What is Needed:

- Dr. Pepper (2/3 cup)
- Ketchup (1 cup)
- Bourbon (2 tbsp.)
- Brown sugar (2 tbsp.)
- Salt (.125 tsp.)
- BBQ seasoning (4 tsp.)
- Worcestershire sauce (1 tbsp.)
- Optional: Celery salt (.25 tsp.)
- Chicken drumsticks (12)

Preparation Method:

1. Combine the sauce fixings (up to the line) in a saucepan. Add the celery salt as desired. Wait for it to boil and adjust the temperature setting to simmer, uncovered, for eight to ten minutes or until slightly thickened, stirring often.
2. On an oiled grill using the med-low temperature setting, cook the chicken, covered for 15 minutes. Turn and continue to grill 15-20 minutes until an internal thermometer reads 170°-175° Fahrenheit. Brush it occasionally with sauce.

Grilled Lemon Chicken

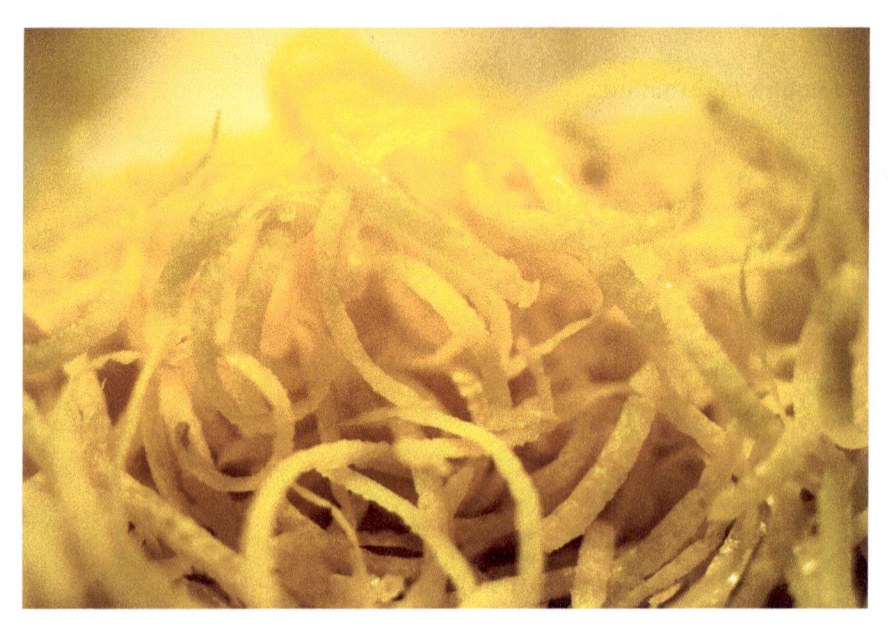

Servings Provided: 12

Time Required: 45 minutes

What is Needed:

- Fryer/broiler chickens - cut up (3-3.5 lb. each)
- Lemonade concentrate - thawed (.75 cup)
- Soy sauce (.33 cup)
- Garlic (1 clove)
- Seasoned salt (1 tsp.)
- Garlic powder (.125 tsp.)
- Celery salt (.5 tsp.)

Preparation Method:

1. Mince the garlic and mix all of the fixings except for the pieces of chicken.
2. Pour half of the mixture into a shallow glass dish. Use a layer of foil or plastic to cover the bowl and place the rest of the lemonade mixture in the fridge.
3. Dip the chicken into lemonade mixture, turning to coat and trash the used marinade.
4. Grill the chicken, covered, using the medium-temperature setting for 30 minutes, turning occasionally. Brush with the reserved lemonade mixture.
5. Grill it for another 10-20 minutes, frequently basting, until a thermometer reads 165° Fahrenheit.

Ground Turkey Burgers

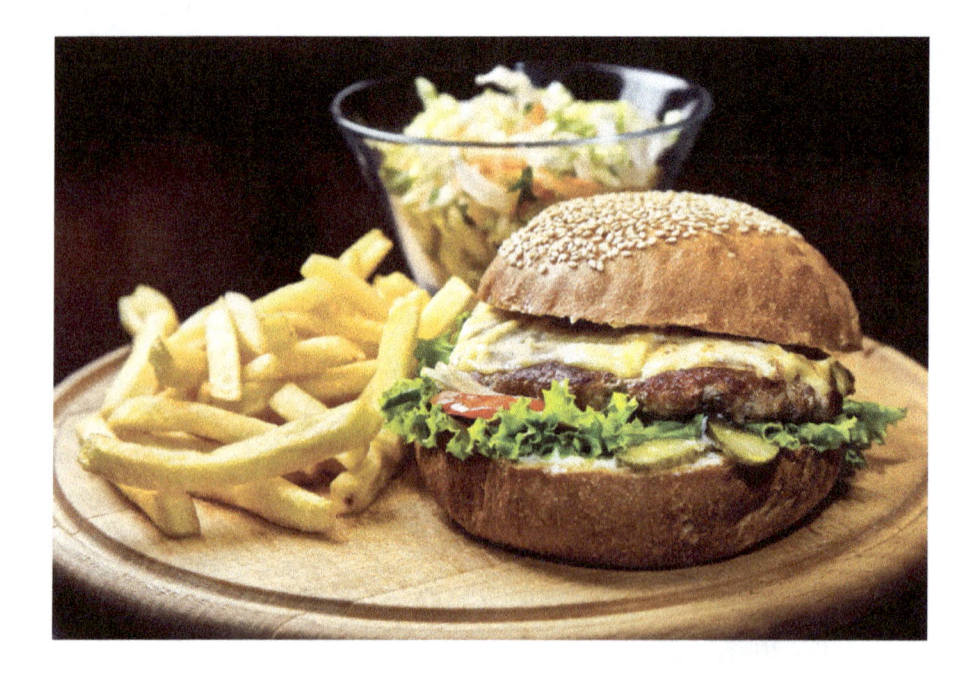

Servings Provided: 6

Time Required: 30 minutes

What is Needed:

- Whisked egg (1 large)
- Whole wheat breadcrumbs (2/3 cup)
- Celery (.5 cup)
- Onion (.25 cup)
- Freshly minced parsley (1 tbsp.)

- Worcestershire sauce (1 tsp.)
- Pepper (.25 tsp)
- Salt (.5 tsp.)
- Dried oregano (1 tsp.)
- Lean ground turkey (1.25 lb.)
- Split whole wheat burger buns (6 whole)

Preparation Method:

1. Chop the onion and celery.
2. Combine the breadcrumbs, egg, celery, seasonings, onion, parsley, and Worcestershire sauce.
3. Add the turkey and shape into patties.
4. Prepare on the grill using the medium-temperature setting until they reach an internal temp of 165° Fahrenheit.
5. Serve the burgers on the buns as desired.

Spiced Chicken With Cilantro Lime Butter

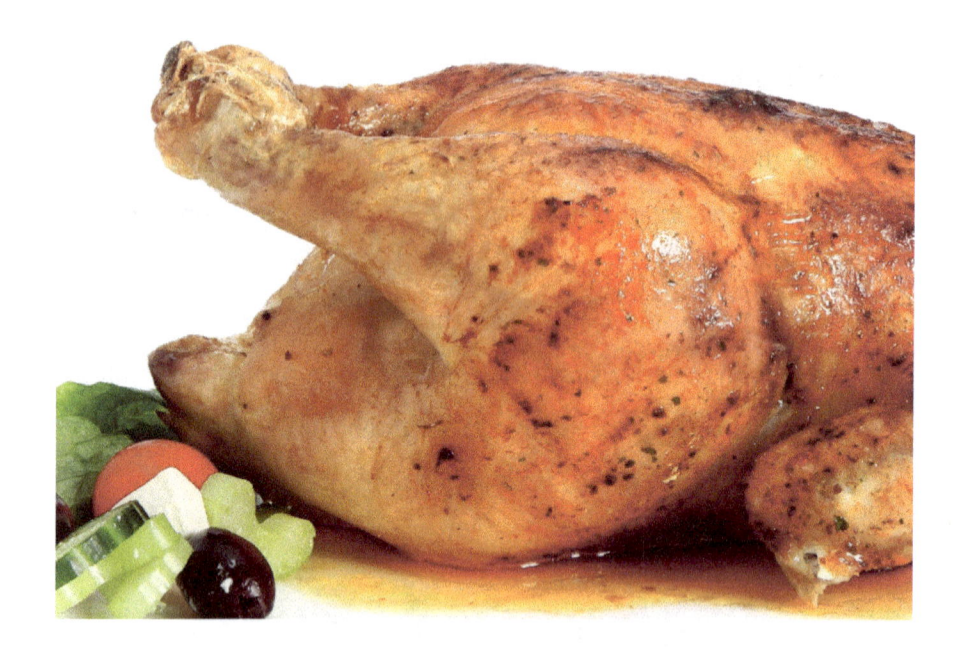

Servings Provided: 6

Time Required: 55 minutes

What is Needed:

   The Sauce Ingredients:

- Chili powder (1 tbsp.)
- Ground cinnamon (2 tsp.)
- Brown sugar (1 tbsp.)
- Baking cocoa (1 tsp.)
- Balsamic vinegar (1 tbsp.)
- Pepper & salt (.5 tsp. each)
- Olive oil (3 tbsp.)
- Bone-in breast halves (6 @ 8 oz. each)

The Lime Butter:

- Melted butter (.33 cup)
- Cilantro (.25 cup)
- Red onion (2 tbsp.)
- Serrano pepper (1)
- Black pepper (.125 tsp.)
- Lime juice (1 tbsp.)

Preparation Method:

1. Finely chop the cilantro, onion, and serrano pepper.
2. Combine the sauce fixings; brown sugar, chili powder, cinnamon, cocoa, pepper, salt, vinegar, and oil. Brush the mixture over chicken.
3. Arrange the chicken skin-side down on the grill rack.
4. Grill the chicken - covered for 15 minutes (indirect medium heat).
5. Flip it over and continue to grill for 20-25 minutes longer (internal temp of 165 °Fahrenheit.
6. Combine the butter fixings to drizzle over the chicken before

serving.

Turkey Pepper Kabobs

Servings Provided: 4

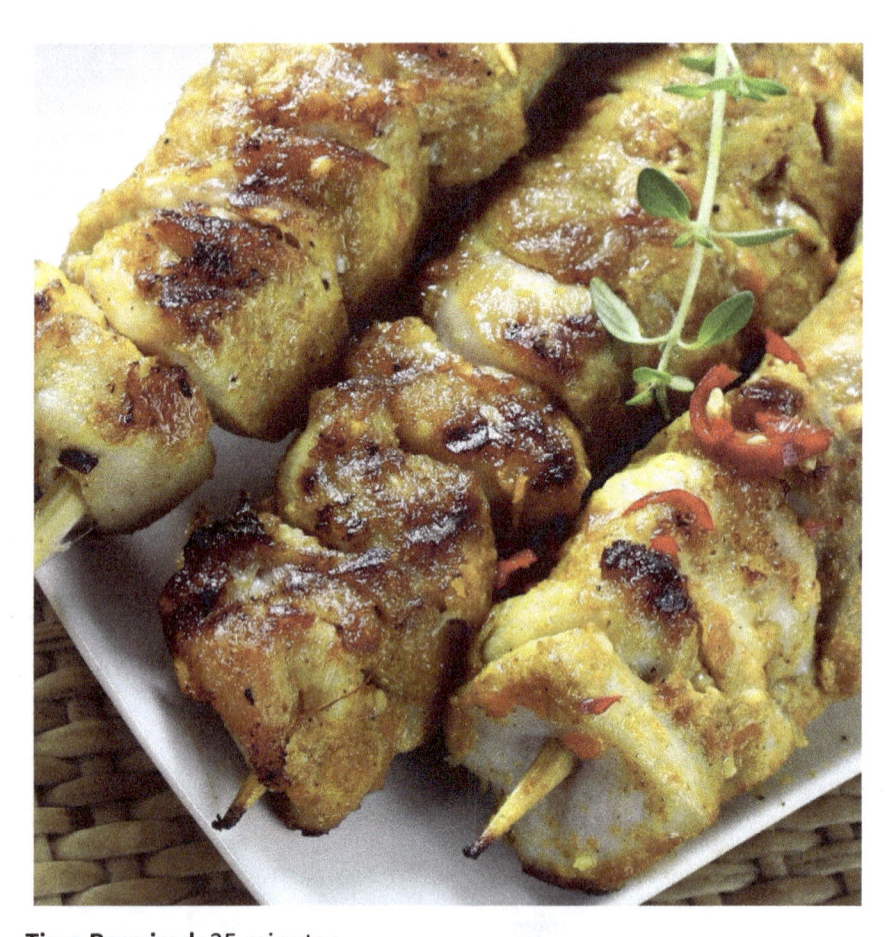

Time Required: 25 minutes

What is Needed:

- Unsweetened pineapple chunks (8 oz. can)

- Brown sugar (.25 cup - packed)
- Worcestershire sauce (2 tbsp.)
- Canola oil (2 tbsp.)
- Garlic (1 clove)
- Prepared mustard (1 tsp.)
- Turkey breast tenderloins (1 lb.)
- Green pepper (1 large)
- Sweet onion (1 large - 0.75-inch pieces)
- Red sweet pepper (1 large)

Preparation Method:

1. Chop the turkey and sweet peppers into one-inch pieces.
2. Drain the pineapple, saving ¼ cup of the juice.
3. Prepare the marinade by mixing the brown sugar with the oil, mustard, Worcestershire sauce, minced garlic, and reserved juice.
4. In another mixing container, cube and toss in the turkey with 1/3 cup of marinade. Refrigerate it covered for two to three hours. Cover and refrigerate the rest of the marinade.
5. On eight soaked wooden skewers or metal, alternately thread the turkey, veggies, and pineapple chunks. Discard the remaining marinade.
6. Arrange the kabobs on an oiled grill rack using medium heat. Grill, covered, until the turkey is no longer pink (8-10 min.), turning occasionally

7. Note: Baste them frequently with the reserved marinade during the last three minutes.

Chapter 4: Beef

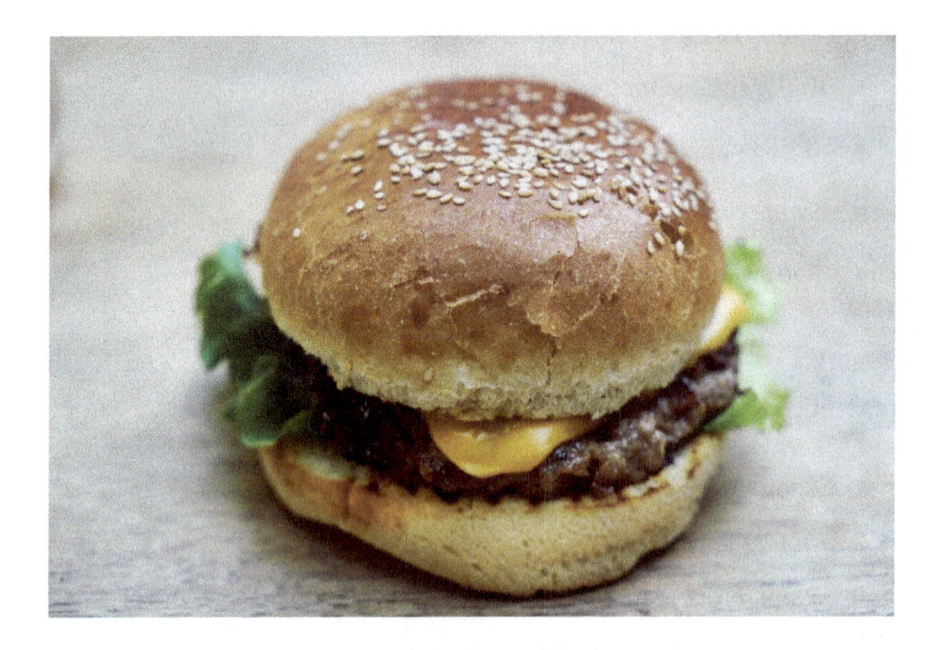

Classic Beef Cheeseburgers

Servings Provided: 4

Time Required: 30 minutes

What is Needed:

- 90% lean ground beef (1 lb.)
- Steak seasoning blend (1.5 tsp.)

- Burger buns (4 - split)
- American/Cheddar/Swiss cheese (4 slices)
- Lettuce (4 leaves)
- Tomato (4 slices)

    Optional Toppings:

- Mustard
- Ketchup
- Onion slices
- Pickle slices

Preparation Method:

1. Prepare the grill until it reaches medium ash-covered coals.
2. While it heats, mix the beef and steak seasoning in a large mixing container, shaping it into four ½-inch thick patties.
3. Arrange the patties on the grid over the coals. Grill the burgers covered for 8 to 10 minutes (for a gas grill 7-9 min.), occasionally turning until an instant-read thermometer inserted horizontally into its center registers at 160° Fahrenheit.
4. About two minutes before the burgers are done, arrange the buns, cut side down, on the grid. Grill until lightly toasted. During the last minute of grilling, top each burger with a slice of cheese to melt.
5. Line the bottom of each bun with lettuce, topping it with the burger, tomato, and chosen toppings. Close the sandwiches and serve.

Grilled Skirt Steak With Peppers & Onions

Servings Provided: 6

Time Required: 50 minutes

What is Needed:

- Apple juice (.5 cup)
- Red wine vinegar (.5 cup)
- Yellow/white onion (.25 cup)
- Rubbed sage (2 tbsp.)
- Ground mustard (3 tsp.)
- Salt (1 tsp.)
- Ground coriander (3 tsp.)
- Black pepper (3 tsp.)
- Garlic clove (1 minced)
- Olive oil (1 cup)
- Beef skirt steak (1.5 lb.)
- Red onions (2 medium)
- Sweet red peppers (2 medium)
- Green onions (12)

Preparation Method:

1. Finely chop the onion, slice the peppers into halves, and trim the green onions. Cut the steak into 5-inch pieces and slice the red onions into ½-in slices.
2. Whisk the first nine ingredients (up to the line) until blended.
3. Slowly whisk in oil. Pour 1.5 cups of the marinade into a large resealable plastic bag. Toss in the beef and seal the bag - tossing it to coat. Refrigerate it overnight. Also, cover and refrigerate the rest of the marinade.
4. Toss the rest of the veggies with ¼ cup of the reserved marinade. Grill the red onions and peppers, covered, using the medium temperature setting (4-6 min. per side)until tender. Grill the green onions one to two minutes until tender.
5. Drain the beef, and trash the marinade in the bag.
6. Grill the beef covered using medium heat (4-6 min. per side) until the meat reaches desired doneness (for medium-rare, a thermometer should read 135° Fahrenheit; medium, 140° Fahrenheit; medium-well, 145° Fahrenheit). Baste with the remaining marinade during the last four minutes of cooking. Let the steak stand for five minutes.
7. Chop the veggies into small pieces and transfer them into an over-sized mixing container. Slice the steak diagonally across the grain into thin slices, add to vegetables, and toss to combine.
8. Serve and enjoy it when it's ready.

Tangy Lime Top Round Steak

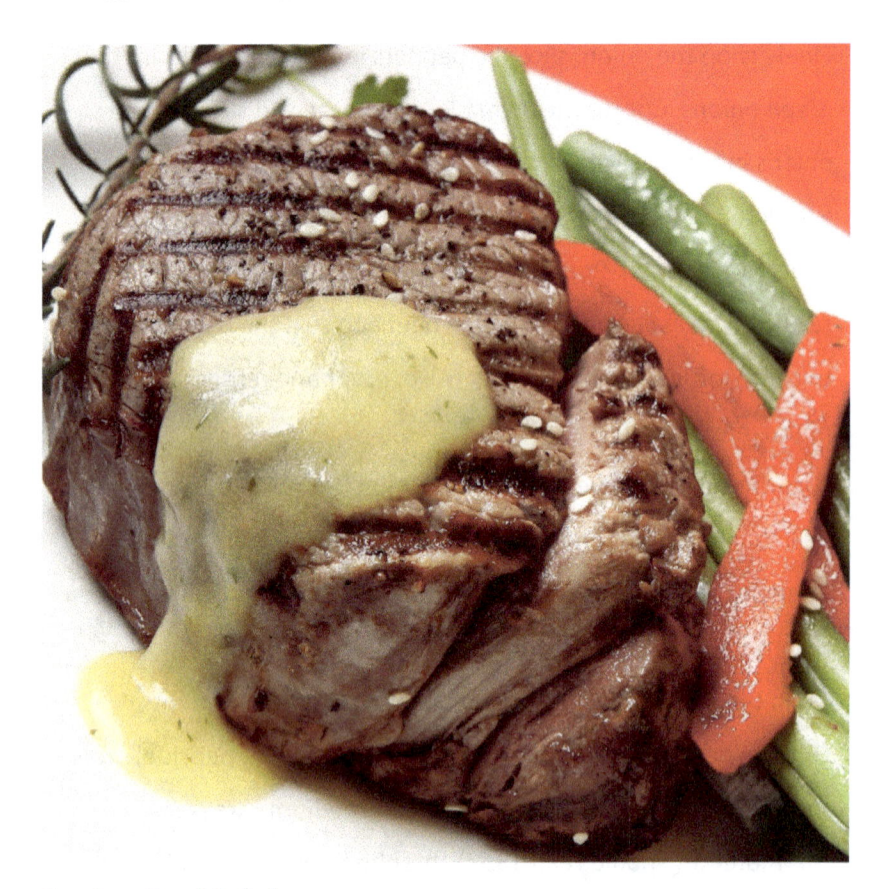

Servings Provided: 4

Time Required: 25 minutes

What is Needed:

- Top round steak (1 lb.)
- Fresh lime juice (.25 cup)
- Worcestershire sauce (1 tbsp.)
- Brown sugar - lightly packed (2 tbsp.)
- Vegetable oil (2 tbsp.)
- Garlic (1 tbsp. - minced)

Preparation Method:

1. Whisk the juice, sugar, oil, Worcestershire, and minced garlic in a small mixing container.
2. Trim the steak, slicing it to a ¾-inch thickness.
3. Place the steak and lime mixture in a zipper-type plastic bag; toss the steak to coat. Securely close the bag and marinate in the fridge for six hours or overnight - turning intermittently.
4. Trash the marinade and place the steak on the grill grid using medium ash-covered coals.
5. Grill, covered for 10-11 minutes, turning occasionally. Don't overcook it. (For medium-rare: 145° Fahrenheit internal temp.)
6. Carve the steak into thin slices.

Whiskey Cheddar Burgers

Servings Provided: 8

Time Required: 30 minutes

What is Needed:

- Whiskey (.25 cup)
- Soy sauce (1 tbsp.)
- Black pepper and salt (.5 tsp. each)
- Worcestershire sauce (1 tbsp.)

- Shredded sharp cheddar cheese (1 cup)
- Onion (.25 cup)
- Seasoned breadcrumbs (2 tbsp.)
- Cloves of garlic (3)
- Paprika (.5 tsp.)
- Dried basil (.5 tsp.)
- Lean ground beef (1.5 lb.)
- Onion/burger buns - split (8)

Optional Toppings:

- Lettuce
- Sliced tomatoes
- BBQ sauce
- Cheddar cheese slices

Preparation Method:

1. Finely chop the onions and cloves. Combine all of the fixings, adding the beef, last.
2. Thoroughly, but gently, combine the mix shaping it into eight ½-inch-thick patties.
3. Prepare a greased grill, using the medium temperature setting.
4. Cook the burgers, covered, for four to five minutes on each side or until a thermometer reads 160° Fahrenheit (internally).
5. Serve the burgers on rolls with toppings as desired.

Chapter 5: Dessert

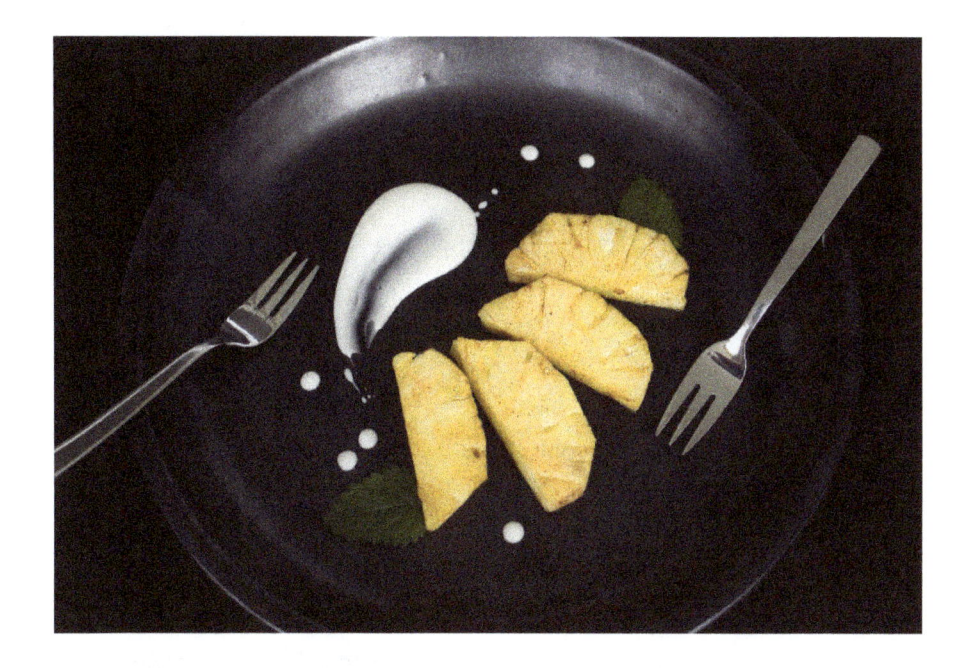

Grilled Pineapple With Lime Dip

Servings Provided: 8

Time Required: 30 minutes

What is Needed:

- Fresh pineapple (1)
- Lime juice (2 tbsp.)
- Packed brown sugar (.25 cup)
- Honey (3 tbsp.)

The Dip:

- Grated lime zest (1 tsp.)
- Brown sugar (1 tbsp.)
- Lime juice (1 tbsp.)
- Honey (2 tbsp.)
- Unchilled cream cheese (3 oz.)
- Plain yogurt (.25 cup)

Preparation Method:

1. Spritz the grill rack using a cooking oil spray before warming the grill. Peel and core the pineapple and slice it vertically into eight wedges. Cut each wedge horizontally into two spears.
2. Combine the honey, brown sugar, and lime juice in a shallow dish and add the pineapple. Toss it and cover to refrigerate for one hour.
3. Beat cream cheese until smooth. Mix in the yogurt with the honey, brown sugar, lime juice, and zest. Cover and pop it into the fridge until it's time to serve.
4. Drain the pineapple, discarding marinade. Grill the pineapple spears using the medium temperature setting (lid on) for three to four minutes per side or until they have grill marks that are golden brown. Serve with the lime dip.

Take Care Of Your Grill!

How to Clean the Grill:

1. Gather a few folded paper towels. Use a large pair of tongs and a high smoke point oil (ex. peanut, sunflower, canola). Olive oil will work in a pinch.
2. Dip the paper towels into a portion of the chosen oil and run it across the grates at least three times to create a non-stick surface to help prevent the meat or fish from breaking during the cooking process.
3. Easy - yet healthy!

PART VI

Chapter 1: Easy Recipes for Managing Kidney Problems

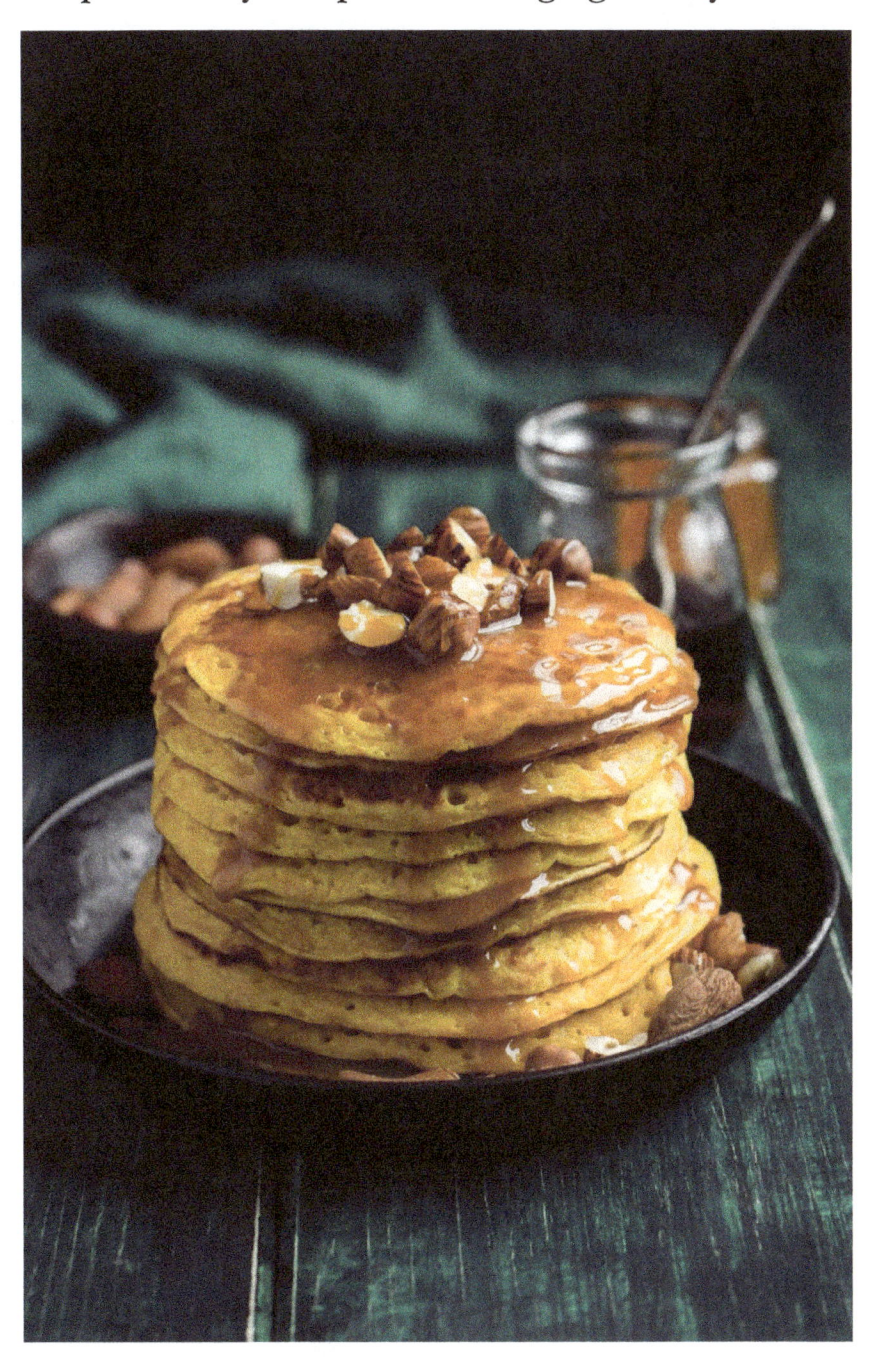

Pumpkin Pancakes

Total Prep & Cooking Time: 40 minutes

Yields: 2 servings

Nutrition Facts: Calories: 183 | Carbs: 39g | Protein: 5.4g | Fat: 1.2g | Sodium: 130mg

Ingredients:

- Two egg whites
- Two tsps. of pumpkin pie spice
- One tsp. of baking powder
- One tbsp. of brown sugar
- Three packets of Stevia
- 1.25 cups of all-purpose flour
- Two cups each of
  - Rice milk
  - Salt-free pumpkin puree

Method:

1. Start by mixing all the dry ingredients together in a bowl – baking powder, Stevia, sugar, flour, and pumpkin pie spice.

2. Now, take another bowl and, in it, mix the rice milk and pumpkin puree thoroughly.

3. In another bowl, form stiff peaks by whipping egg whites.

4. Take the mixture of dry ingredients and add them to the wet ingredients. Blend them in. Once you get a smooth mixture, add the egg whites, and whip them.

5. Grill the mixture on an oiled griddle on medium flame.

6. When you notice bubbles forming on the pancakes, you have to flip them.

7. Cook both sides of the pancakes evenly so that they turn golden brown.

Pasta Salad

Total Prep & Cooking Time: 50 minutes

Yields: 4 servings (half a cup each serving)

Nutrition Facts: Calories: 69 | Carbs: 12.5g | Protein: 2.5g | Fat: 1.3g | Sodium: 72mg

Ingredients:

- A quarter cup of olives (sliced after being pitted)
- One cup of chopped cauliflower
- Two cups of fusilli pasta (cooked)
- Half a unit each of
  - Green bell pepper (sliced)
  - Red onion (chopped)
  - Tomato (small-sized, diced)

Method:

1. Start by cooking the pasta, and for that, you have to follow the directions as mentioned on the package.
2. Now, drain the pasta. Add all the vegetables.
3. Choose any dressing of your choice, but it has to be low-fat. Toss the pasta and the veggies in the dressing.
4. Serve and enjoy!

Broccoli and Apple Salad

Total Prep & Cooking Time: 15 minutes

Yields: 8 servings (3/4 cup each serving)

Nutrition Facts: Calories: 160 | Carbs: 18g | Protein: 4g | Fat: 8g | Sodium: 63mg

Ingredients:

- Four cups of fresh florets of broccoli
- One medium-sized apple
- Half a cup each of
    - Sweetened cranberries (dried)
    - Red onion
- A quarter cup each of
    - Walnuts
    - Fresh parsley
    - Mayonnaise
- Two tbsps. each of
    - Apple cider vinegar
    - Honey
- A three-fourth cup of plain Greek yogurt (low-fat)

Method:

1. Prepare the broccoli florets by cutting into bite-sized chunks. Trim them properly. Take the apple and cut into small pieces as well but in the unpeeled state. Prepare the parsley by chopping them coarsely.

2. Now, take a large-sized bowl and add the mayonnaise, yogurt, vinegar, honey, and parsley. Whisk them together.

3. Take the remaining ingredients and add them too. Make sure they are evenly coated with the yogurt mixture. Once prepared, keep the salad in the refrigerator because it is best served when chilled. It allows the flavors to combine properly. Before serving, stir the salad.

Notes:

- *You can use your favorite type of apple.*
- *If you want, you can sprinkle some more parsley on top just before serving.*

Pineapple Frangelico Sorbet

Total Prep & Cooking Time: 2 hours 10 minutes

Yields: 4 servings

Nutrition Facts: Calories: 119 | Carbs: 28g | Protein: 1g | Fat: 0.2g | Sodium: 2.4mg

Ingredients:

- Two tsps. of Stevia
- One tbsp. of Frangelico (keep two tsps. extra)
- Half a cup of unsweetened pineapple juice
- Two cups of pineapple (fresh)

Method:

1. Take all the ingredients in the container of the blender and process them until you get a smooth mixture.
2. Then, take this mixture and divide it into ice cubes. Keep it in the refrigerator and allow it to freeze.
3. When you find that the mixture has frozen, take them out and blend them in the food processor again. This process will give you a fluffy texture.
4. Before you serve, refreeze the sorbet.

Egg Muffins

Total Prep & Cooking Time: 45 minutes

Yields: 8 servings

Nutrition Facts: Calories: 154 | Carbs: 3g | Protein: 12g | Fat: 10g | Sodium: 155mg

Ingredients:

- Half an lb. of ground pork
- Half a tsp. of herb seasoning blend of your choice
- A quarter tsp. of salt
- Eight eggs (large-sized)
- A quarter tsp. each of
    - Onion powder
    - Garlic powder
    - Poultry seasoning
- One cup each of
    - Onion
    - Bell peppers (A mixture of orange, yellow, and red)

Method:

1. Set the oven temperature to 350 degrees F and use cooking spray to coat a muffin tin of regular size.

2. Prepare the onions and bell peppers by dicing them finely.

3. Take a bowl and in it, combine the following ingredients – garlic powder, poultry seasoning, pork, onion powder, and herb seasoning blend. Form the sausage by combining all of this properly.

4. Now cook the sausage in a non-stick skillet. Once it has been appropriately cooked, drain the sausage.

5. Use salt and milk substitute/milk to beat the eggs in a bowl. In it, add the veggies and the sausage mix.

6. Take the prepared muffin tin and pour the egg mixture into it. You have to leave enough space for the muffins so that they can rise. Bake them for about 20-22 minutes.

Notes: *If there are extra muffins, then you can have them as a quick breakfast the next day, and you simply have to reheat them for about 40 seconds.*

Linguine With Broccoli, Chickpeas, and Ricotta

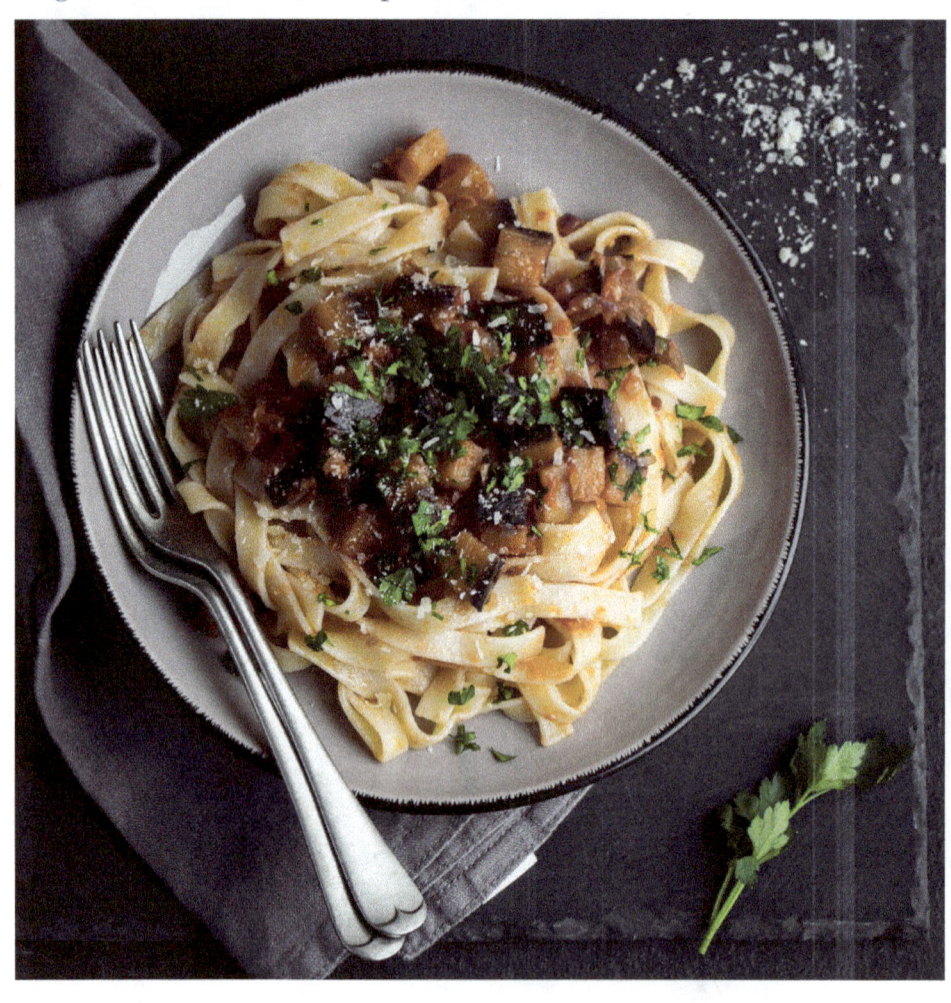

Total Prep & Cooking Time: 1 hour 5 minutes

Yields: 4 servings

Nutrition Facts: Calories: 404 | Carbs: 49.8g | Protein: 13.2g | Fat: 17.5g | Sodium: 180.4mg

Ingredients:

- Eight ounces of ricotta cheese that have been kept at room temperature
- A bunch of Tuscan kale (chopped into bite-sized chunks and stemmed)
- One-third cup of extra-virgin olive oil
- A pinch of black pepper
- Two cloves of garlic (sliced thinly)
- Fourteen ounces of chickpeas (rinsed after draining)
- Twelve ounces of spaghetti or linguine pasta
- A pinch of kosher salt
- One lemon
- Half a teaspoon of red pepper flakes
- Two tablespoons of unsalted butter
- To taste – Flaky sea salt

Method:

1. Take a large pot and add water to it. Add salt and bring the water to a boil. Cook the pasta by following the directions mentioned on the package. They must be perfectly al dente. Once the pasta is done, you have to drain it but, at the same time, reserve half a cup of the cooking water.

2. Heat the broiler and adjust the rack. Toss the following ingredients together in a bowl – garlic, chickpeas, broccoli, one-third cup of oil, and

red pepper flakes. Everything should become evenly coated. Use pepper and salt to season the mixture.

3. Take a sheet pan and spread the mixture out on it evenly.

4. Take the kale and add it to the previous bowl you used. Toss it again along with the remaining oil, if any. If you need it, then you can drizzle some more oil on top. Spread the kale in a second sheet pan in an even layer.

5. You have to take one sheet at a time while working. Broil the chickpeas and broccoli and halfway through the process, toss them. The broccoli should become charred and tender, and the chickpeas should be toasty. It will take about seven minutes. Then, broil the kale too for about five minutes, and they should become crispy.

6. Take the lemon, zest it, and then cut it into two halves. Take one half and form four wedges out of it. The juice of the lemon will have to be squeezed out on the roasted veggies and then use pepper and salt to season.

7. Place the pasta back in the pot. Take the pasta water you had earlier reserved and add it to the pasta and the lemon zest, butter, and ricotta. Keep tossing so that everything is well incorporated. Now, add the roasted veggies too. If you need, add some more pasta water while tossing.

8. Now, your linguine is done, and you have to divide it among four bowls—season with pepper and flaky sea salt. Squeeze a few drops of lemon on top and serve. If you want, drizzle some more oil before serving.

Ground Beef Soup

Total Prep & Cooking Time: 35 minutes

Yields: 6 servings

Nutrition Facts: Calories: 222 | Carbs: 19g | Protein: 20g | Fat: 8g | Sodium: 170mg

Ingredients:

- Half a cup of onion
- One tbsp. of sour cream
- Three cups of mixed vegetables (frozen, peas, green beans, corn, and carrots)
- One-third cup of uncooked white rice
- Two cups of water
- One cup of beef broth (reduced-sodium variety)
- One tsp. of browning sauce and seasoning of your choice
- Two tsps. of lemon pepper seasoning of your choice
- One lb. of ground beef (lean)

Method:

1. Prepare the onion by chopping them thoroughly. Then, take a large-sized saucepan and, in it, brown the onion and ground beef together. Drain the juices and excess fat.

2. Add the browning sauce and seasonings. Then, add the mixed veggies, rice, water, and beef broth and mix everything together.

3. Bring the mixture to a boil after placing it on high flame. Once the mixture starts boiling, reduce the flame to medium-low and cover the saucepan. Allow it to simmer and cook it for half an hour.

4. Once done, remove the pan from the flame and add the sour cream. Stir it in and serve.

Apple Oatmeal Crisp

Total Prep & Cooking Time: 40 minutes

Yields: 8 servings

Nutrition Facts: Calories: 297 | Carbs: 42g | Protein: 3g | Fat: 13g | Sodium: 95mg

Ingredients:

- A three-quarter cup of brown sugar
- Half a cup of butter
- One tsp. of cinnamon
- Half a cup of all-purpose flour
- Five apples (if possible, then Granny Smith ones)
- One cup of whole oatmeal

Method:

1. Set the temperature of the oven to 350 degrees F and preheat. Peel the apples, core them, and then cut them into slices.

2. Take a bowl and then mix the following ingredients in it together – brown sugar, oatmeal, cinnamon, and flour.

3. Use a pastry cutter to cut the butter into the oatmeal and make sure they are well blended.

4. Take a baking pan of 9 by 9 inches in size and place the sliced apples in it.

5. Take the oatmeal mixture and sprinkle it on top of the apples.

6. Bake the mixture for about thirty to thirty-five minutes.

Chapter 2: Weekend Recipes for Renal Diet

Hawaiian Chicken Salad Sandwich

Total Prep & Cooking Time: 10 minutes + chilling

Yields: 4 servings

Nutrition Facts: Calories: 349 | Carbs: 24g | Protein: 22g | Fat: 17g | Sodium: 398mg

Ingredients:

- One cup of pineapple tidbits
- Two cups of cooked chicken
- One-third cup of carrots
- Half a cup each of
    - Green bell pepper
    - Mayonnaise (low-fat)
- Four units of flatbread
- Half a tsp. of black pepper

Method:

1. Take the cooked chicken and chop it into bite-sized pieces.
2. Prepare the pineapple by draining it and then shred the carrots and chop the bell pepper.
3. Take all the ingredients in a medium-sized bowl and mix them well.
4. Refrigerate the mixture until it is thoroughly chilled.
5. Before serving, spread the chicken on the flatbread's open surface, or if you prefer it wrapped, you can use a tortilla too.

Apple Puffs

Total Prep & Cooking Time: 1 hour 20 minutes

Yields: 12 servings

Nutrition Facts: Calories: 156 | Carbs: 22g | Protein: 1.5g | Fat: 7.3g | Sodium: 176mg

Ingredients:

- Eight ounces of puff dough sheets
- One can (21 oz.) of apple pie filling
- Half a tsp. of rum extract
- One tsp. each of
    - Powdered sugar
    - Baking soda
    - Ground cinnamon

Method:

1. First, you have to thaw the puff dough sheets at room temperature, and it will take you approximately 1 hour.

2. Set the temperature of the oven to 400 degrees F and preheat.

3. Take a bowl, and in it, add the apple pie filling. If you have already sliced the apples, then you can form thirds from them now. Mix the rum extract and cinnamon with the apples.

4. Once the dough has been completely thawed, take one of the sheets and cut nine equal squares from it. Take the other sheet, and you will need only one-third of it to cut another three such squares.

5. Now, take the muffin tin and place the squares in each of the tins. In each of these squares, spoon some of the apple mixture.

6. Bake the preparation in the preheated oven for fifteen minutes, and they should become golden brown in color.

7. Once done, remove the puffs from the muffin tins and before serving, sprinkle some powdered sugar on top of each apple puff. Serve them warm.

Creamy Orzo and Vegetables

Total Prep & Cooking Time: 30 minutes

Yields: 6 servings

Nutrition Facts: Calories: 176 | Carbs: 25g | Protein: 10g | Fat: 4g | Sodium: 193mg

Ingredients:

- Half a cup of frozen green peas
- One tsp. of curry powder
- One carrot (medium-sized)
- One zucchini (small-sized)
- One onion (small-sized)
- One clove of garlic
- Three cups of chicken broth (low-sodium variety)

- Two tbsps. each of
  - Olive oil
  - Fresh parsley
- A quarter tsp. of black pepper
- A quarter cup of Parmesan cheese (freshly grated)
- One cup of cooked orzo pasta
- A quarter tsp. of salt

Method:

1. Start by preparing the veggies. Chop the zucchini and onion. Chop the garlic finely. Then, take the carrots and shred them.

2. Place a large-sized skillet on the oven over medium flame. Heat olive oil in the skillet. Sauté the following ingredients in it for about five minutes – carrots, zucchini, onion, and garlic.

3. After that, add the curry powder to the mixture. Season with salt and then add the chicken broth. Bring the mixture to a boil.

4. Now, add the cooked orzo pasta and keep stirring until the mixture starts boiling. Cover the skillet and allow the mixture to simmer. Keep stirring from time to time and cook the pasta for another 10 minutes. By this time, the pasta will become al dente, and the liquid will be absorbed.

5. Add the chopped parsley, cheese, and the frozen peas into the pasta. Keep heating until the vegetables are sufficiently hot, and if you want to enhance the creaminess, then you can add some more broth—season with pepper.

Minestrone Soup

Total Prep & Cooking Time: 45 minutes

Yields: 4 servings

Nutrition Facts: Calories: 144 | Carbs: 21.9g | Protein: 5.9g | Fat: 4.3g | Sodium: 55.1mg

Ingredients:

- Four cups of low-sodium chicken broth (low-fat)
- One carrot (large-sized)
- One and a half cups of dry macaroni (elbow-shaped)
- 14 oz. of tomatoes (diced, without any salt content)
- Two stalks of celery
- Two garlic cloves
- Half a cup of zucchini (freshly chopped)
- One teaspoon each of
    - Dried basil
    - Dried oregano
    - Freshly ground black pepper
- Half an onion (large-sized)
- One can of green snap beans (without any salt content)
- Two tbsps. of olive oil

Method:

1. Prepare the veggies by dicing zucchini, garlic, and onion. Then, take the carrots and shred them. Either use fresh green beans or canned ones, but you have to cut them into pieces of half an inch size.

2. Take a Dutch oven or a large pot and place it on medium flame—heat olive oil in the pot. Add the diced onions in the pot as well and then cook them for a couple of minutes until they become translucent.

3. Add zucchini, carrot, celery, and garlic, and if you are using fresh green beans, then add them too. Cook the vegetables for about five minutes and they will become tender.

4. Add black pepper, oregano, basil, and if you are using canned beans, then add them now.

5. Add the chicken broth and the diced tomatoes and keep stirring.

6. Bring the mixture to a boil and once it starts boiling, allow the mixture to simmer for about ten minutes.

7. Add the pasta and cook them for an additional ten minutes by following the directions mentioned on the package.

8. Before serving, garnish the pasta with fresh basil on top. Serve into bowls and enjoy!

Frosted Grapes

Total Prep & Cooking Time: 1 hour 5 minutes

Yields: 10 servings (serving size – half a cup)

Nutrition Facts: Calories: 88 | Carbs: 21g | Protein: 1g | Fat: 0g | Sodium: 41mg

Ingredients:

- Three oz. of flavored gelatin
- Five cups of seedless grapes

Method:

1. De-steam the seedless grapes after you have washed them. After that, let them be but make sure they are slightly damp.
2. In a large-sized bowl, add the dry gelatin mix. Remember that you shouldn't be pouring in water.
3. Add these damp grapes into the bowl, and in order to coat them uniformly, toss them well.
4. Now, take a baking sheet, and place these grapes on the sheet in an even layer.
5. Freeze them for 1 hour and then serve chilled.

Notes: *The flavor of the gelatin you use can be adjusted as per your choice. If you want to decrease the carbs, then use gelatin that is sugar-free.*

Yogurt and Fruit Salad

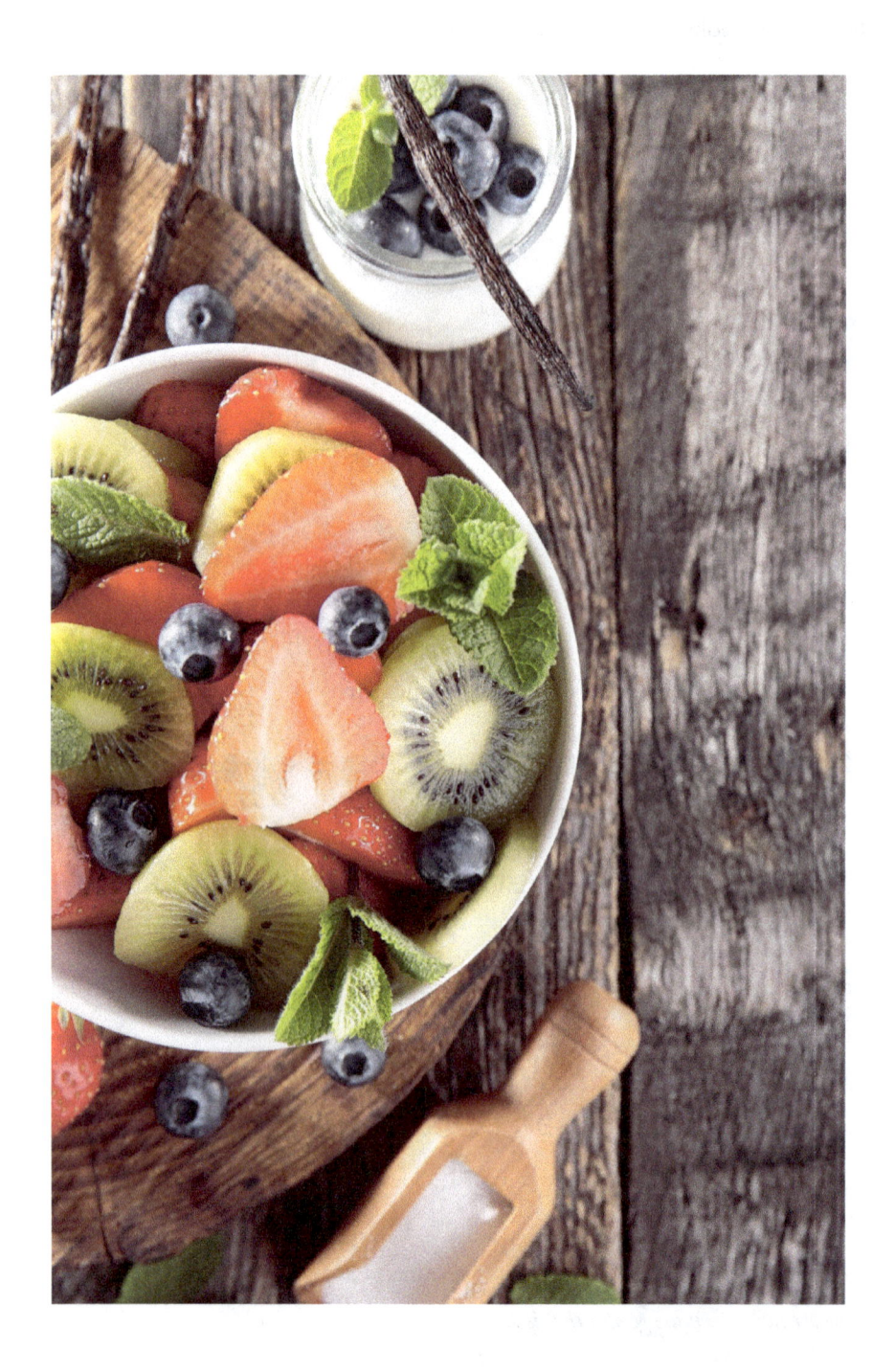

Total Prep & Cooking Time: 2 hours 20 minutes

Yields: 4 servings

Nutrition Facts: Calories: 99 | Carbs: 22g | Protein: 2.6g | Fat: 0.7g | Sodium: 12mg

Ingredients:

- One-third cup of dried cranberries
- Half a cup of pineapple chunks (fresh)
- Six strawberries (large-sized)
- Six ounces of Greek yogurt (strawberry flavored)
- Four ounces of mandarin oranges (drained, light syrup)
- Ten green grapes
- One apple (with skin, medium-sized)

Method:

1. Wash the strawberries, grapes, and apples. After that, pat them dry.
2. Slice the apples and chop them into bite-sized chunks.
3. Then, take the strawberries and slice them as well.
4. Mix the following ingredients together – yogurt, dried cranberries, pineapple, Mandarin oranges, grapes, and apples.
5. Keep the mixture covered and put it in the refrigerator for two hours.
6. Before serving, garnish the preparation with sliced strawberries.

Beet and Apple Juice Blend

Total Prep & Cooking Time: 5 minutes

Yields: 2 servings

Nutrition Facts: Calories: 53 | Carbs: 13g | Protein: 1g | Fat: 0g | Sodium: 66mg

Ingredients:

- A quarter cup of parsley
- Half a beet (medium-sized)
- Half an apple (medium-sized)
- One carrot (fresh, medium-sized)
- One stalk of celery

Method:

1. Process the following ingredients together in a juicer – parsley, celery, carrot, beet, and apple.
2. Take the mixture and pour it into two small glasses. You can either keep the juice in the refrigerator to chill or have it right away.

Notes: *Even though juices are healthy, for kidney patients, you have to be careful so that you don't increase your potassium intake too much.*

Baked Turkey Spring Rolls

Total Prep & Cooking Time: 1 hour 30 minutes

Yields: 8 servings (per serving – 2 spring rolls)

Nutrition Facts: Calories: 197 | Carbs: 9.6g | Protein: 23.3g | Fat: 7.3g | Sodium: 82.2mg

Ingredients:

- 2.5 cups of coleslaw mix
- Two tsps. of freshly ground black pepper
- Twenty ounces of turkey breast (ground)
- Two tbsps. each of
  - Vegetable oil
  - Minced cilantro
- One tbsp. each of
  - Sesame oil
  - Balsamic vinegar
- Two tsps. of freshly ground black pepper
- Sixteen pastry wrappers (frozen spring roll wraps)
- Cooking spray

Method:

1. Set the temperature of the oven to 400 degrees F and preheat.

2. Take the spring roll wrappers out from the freezer so that they can stay under room temperature. Thawing should be done at least half an hour before preparation.

3. Now, take a bowl, and in it, mix the following ingredients with the raw turkey – minced cilantro, sesame oil, and balsamic vinegar.

4. Take a large-sized skillet, and in it, pour two tbsps. of vegetable oil. Put the skillet on medium-high flame and preheat. Add the ground turkey into the skillet and crumble it by stirring. To cook the turkey properly, you have to keep sautéing the mixture.

5. Then, you have to add the mixture of coleslaw to the turkey and keep cooking for another five minutes. Season with freshly ground black pepper – two tsps. should be enough. Mix everything properly.

6. Once done, remove the skillet from the flame. Use a strainer to drain any remaining liquid.

7. Take one spring roll wrapper and near one corner of it – add the filling diagonally. You can take three tbsps. of filling for one roll. There should be adequate space left on both sides. Fold one side towards the inside and do the same with the other side. Roll them and make sure the sights have been tucked in properly. Use water to moisten one of the sides of the wrapper because this helps to seal properly.

8. Take the remaining wrappers and follow the same steps with them.

9. Use non-stick cooking spray to coat the baking pan's base and then place the spring rolls in it. Place the pan in the oven, and it should be complete in half an hour when given at 400 degrees F.

10. You can also serve the rolls with a sweet chili sauce, but this has not been included in the nutrition facts.

Crab-Stuffed Celery Logs

Total Prep & Cooking Time: 10 minutes

Yields: 4 servings

Nutrition Facts: Calories: 34 | Carbs: 2g | Protein: 2g | Fat: 2g | Sodium: 94mg

Ingredients:

- Two tsps. of mayonnaise
- One tbsp. of red onion
- A quarter cup of crab meat
- Four ribs or celery (approx. eight inches in size)
- A quarter tsp. of paprika
- Half a tsp. of lemon juice

Method:

1. Take the celery ribs and trim the ends. Prepare the crab meat by draining it and then use two forks to flake the meat. Chop the onion and mince it thoroughly.

2. Take a small-sized bowl and in it, add the lemon juice, mayonnaise, onion, and crab meat and combine them properly.

3. Take a whole tablespoon full of the mixture and fill the celery rib with it.

4. Each rib of celery has to be cut into three equal pieces.

5. Sprinkle some paprika on top of each of these celery logs.

Couscous Salad

Total Prep & Cooking Time: 50 minutes

Yields: 4 servings (half a cup per serving)

Nutrition Facts: Calories: 151 | Carbs: 28.7g | Protein: 4.9g | Fat: 2.5g | Sodium: 14.3mg

Ingredients:

- One teaspoon each of
    - Dried oregano
    - Allspice
- Two lemons (juiced)
- One tbsp. each of
    - Olive oil
    - Minced garlic
- Half a cup each of
    - Red bell pepper (chopped)
    - Yellow bell pepper (chopped)
    - Carrots (chopped)
    - Frozen corn
- One cup each of
    - Dry couscous
    - Whole sugar snap peas
- Three peeled cucumbers (large-sized)

Method:

1. Follow the package instructions to prepare the couscous. After that, allow it to chill.

2. Take a large bowl and mix the following ingredients: cucumbers, couscous, snow peas, carrots, corn, yellow pepper, and red pepper.

3. Take another bowl of small size and, in it, whisk the following ingredients together – dried oregano, allspice, lemon juice, olive oil, and minced garlic.

4. Combine everything and serve it chilled.

Chapter 3: One-Week Meal Plan

Day 1

Breakfast – Pumpkin Pancakes

Lunch – Ground Beef Soup

Snacks – Frosted Grapes

Dinner – Pasta Salad

Day 2

Breakfast – Yogurt and Fruit Salad

Lunch – Broccoli and Apple Salad

Snacks – Apple Puffs

Dinner – Baked Turkey Spring Rolls

Day 3

Breakfast – Egg Muffins

Lunch – Minestrone Soup

Snacks – Crab-Stuffed Celery Logs

Dinner – Hawaiian Chicken Salad Sandwich

Day 4

Breakfast – Yogurt and Fruit Salad

Lunch – Pasta Salad

Snacks – Apple Puffs

Dinner – Linguine with Broccoli, Chickpeas, and Ricotta

Day 5

Breakfast – Beet and Apple Juice Blend

Lunch – Ground Beef Soup

Snacks – Frosted Grapes

Dinner – Baked Turkey Spring Rolls

Day 6

Breakfast – Pumpkin Pancakes

Lunch – Creamy Orzo and Vegetables

Snacks – Pineapple Frangelico Sorbet

Dinner – Couscous Salad

Day 7

Breakfast – Egg Muffins

Lunch – Broccoli and Apple Salad

Snacks – Pineapple Frangelico Sorbet

Dinner – Ground Beef Soup

CPSIA information can be obtained
at www.ICGtesting.com
Printed in the USA
BVHW011747031120
592432BV00005B/14